CLINICAL PHENOMENOLOGY AND COGNITIVE PSYCHOLOGY

DAVID FEWTRELL AND KIERON O'CONNOR

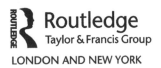

LONDON AND NEW YORK

First published in 1995

Published 2016 by Routledge

This edition first published in 2014
by Routledge
2 Park Square, Milton Park, Abingdon, Oxon, OX14 4RN

Simultaneously published in the USA and Canada
by Routledge
711 Third Avenue, New York, NY 10017

Routledge is an imprint of the Taylor & Francis Group, an informa business

First issued in paperback 2015

British Library Cataloguing in Publication Data
A catalogue record for this book is available from the British Library

ISBN: 978-0-415-85930-1 (hbk)
ISBN: 978-1-138-97095-3 (pbk)

Publisher's Note
The publisher has gone to great lengths to ensure the quality of this reprint but
points out that some imperfections in the original copies may be apparent.

Disclaimer
The publisher has made every effort to trace copyright holders and would
welcome correspondence from those they have been unable to trace.

Clinical phenomenology and cognitive psychology

Cognitive therapies are often biased in their assessment of clinical problems by their emphasis on the role of verbally-mediated thought in shaping our emotions, and in stressing the influence of thought upon feeling. Alternatively, a more phenomenological appraisal of psychological dysfunction suggests that emotion and thinking are complementary processes which influence each other.

Cognitive psychology developed out of information-processing models, whereas phenomenological psychology is rooted in a philosophical perspective which avoids the assumptions of positivist methodology. But, despite their different origins, the two disciplines overlap and complement each other. In *Clinical Phenomenology and Cognitive Psychology* David Fewtrell and Kieron O'Connor illustrate how feeling states are a crucial component of mental health problems and, if adequately differentiated, can result in a greater understanding of mental health. *Clinical Phenomenology and Cognitive Psychology* highlights the impact of self-experience in shaping a variety of common and rare syndromes.

Clinical phenomenology and cognitive psychology

David Fewtrell and Kieron O'Connor

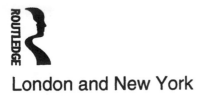

London and New York

This book is dedicated to Mrs E.M. O'Connor and in the memory of Jay Fewtrell. Many thanks to Yvonne-Marianne Fewtrell.

First published 1995
by Routledge
11 New Fetter Lane, London EC4P 4EE

Simultaneously published in the USA and Canada
by Routledge
29 West 35th Street, New York, NY 10001

Typeset in Times by Michael Mepham, Frome, Somerset
Printed and bound in Great Britain
by Biddles Ltd, Guildford and King's Lynn

British Library Cataloguing in Publication Data
A catalogue record for this book is available from the British Library

Library of Congress Cataloging in Publication Data
A catalog record for this book has been requested

ISBN 0–415–06946–7

Contents

Foreword

This book is intended to highlight the realm of conscious experience which anti-subjectivist tendencies in behaviourism, psychophysiology and organic psychiatry have disowned and dismissed from the mental health field. Under the guise of 'empiricism' the issue of conscious experience has been squeezed out of mainstream psychology and into a tight corner, as if an embarrassing irrelevance to 'real' aspects of human functioning. Yet people in distress rarely formulate their problems in diagnostic, behavioural or physiological language spontaneously. As a general rule, it can be said that the distressed use subjectivity as the predominant frame of reference.

The 'objective' constructs of psychological dysfunction are sometimes imposed upon the distressed by their professional helpers. It is crucial to enquire as to what we are being objective about. Although physiological indices record a well-defined phenomenon, and any number of trained judges may agree on the presence and amplitude of such criteria, the criteria fail to reflect the experiential aspects of distress. Therefore criteria reflecting introspective events need to be set within the same frame of reference to the object of study.

Cognitive psychology as a school of psychotherapy has gone some way to acknowledge that covert subjective activity can be rendered amenable to observation and change and that it can be accorded the status of an independent and influential phenomenon. But cognitive psychotherapy is a long way from coming to terms with the complex processes of the psyche and their relation to expressed thought and behaviour. It therefore seems timely to elaborate the cognitive approach by introducing a phenomenological framework to the clinical psychological sciences. This is in order to build upon cognitive therapy by use of observations which phenomenologically minded clinicians have provided over more than a century.

This book is aimed at drawing together some of the observations and concepts of phenomenology and cognitive psychology, with a view to enriching the role of both within the context of psychopathology.

Many field-workers in mental health have heard of the term 'phenomenology', but surprisingly few field-workers are acquainted with its definition. Structural phenomenology is based on a philosophical approach which aims to describe only what can be gleaned from the information available; no more, but importantly, no less. It is therefore a descriptive approach, with no pre-conceived assumptions. This orientation is particularly helpful in highlighting prejudices in clinical interpretation. A phenomenological study of cognition incorporates thought and feeling within its scope. However, phenomenology has never assumed a fixed cause and effect relationship between thought and feeling, in keeping with its role of steering clear of aetiological assumptions and theoretical axioms. In contrast, many cognitive psychotherapists rely heavily upon the assumption that thought is a primary determinant of emotion. In support of this assumption, there is a mounting quantity of evidence that verbal mediation has a direct bearing on prevailing mood. However, there is an alternative hypothesis to the cognitivists' preferred emphasis, outlined recently by Greenberg and Safran (1987), namely that emotion determines the content and nature of thought, rather than the other way round. In reality, thought and feeling interact in a complex way which is bi-directional. For example, it can be demonstrated not only that depression-loaded cognitions lower mood, but also that the lowering of mood has repercussions on further cognitive activity.

Writers with a phenomenological bias have had little direct bearing on the recent psychological literature. Succinct works exemplifying phenomenological principles which appeared during the heyday of behaviourism were considered incompatible with the prevailing philosophical atmosphere of the day. There have been attempts to find common ground between behaviourism and phenomenology (e.g. Watchel 1977) and there are threads of similarity when, for example, each is compared to psychoanalysis. But the gulf created by the phenomenologists' focus on consciousness had remained unbridgeable in the clinical field, until the arrival of recent cognitive therapies. These cognitive approaches, themselves scions of the established behavioural tradition, have sponsored the re-entry of subjective thought and feeling into acceptable parlance. It is likely that we will look back in retrospect to the present era and be thankful to cognitive psychotherapy for rendering internal processes 'respectable' again.

In parallel, the structure and temporal sequence of subjective events have preoccupied clinical phenomenology since its inception, to the extent that in psychopathology, phenomenology has come to be seen as the science of introspection. The scientifically minded among psychologists have tended to avoid the introspective component of psychological activity, for fear it cannot be subjected to hypotheses testing. However, phenomenological description provides information. This type of observation is no less amenable to empirical investigation than behavioural data. Subtlety does not imply inaccessibility, and there are many unresolved problems in psychopathology, both conceptual and clinical, which would profit from detailed consideration of subjects' introspective reports.

The significance of the internal pyschic events which comprise consciousness cannot be negated, whatever theoretical gymnastics are employed to justify their omission. As Karl Popper, R. B. Cattell and others have pointed out, the nature of scientific endeavour (and by implication, the quality) is determined by its content. Empiricism is not synonymous with reductionism. If it were, there would be little room for creative investigation and empirical psychology would rapidly gain the easily acquired distinction of being neat, tidy and irrelevant. To avoid this fate, a shift of emphasis toward the structured study of subjectivity, in the spirit of theoretical agnosticism, is timely. Without such changes in direction, the study of consciousness will become progressively more insubstantial in scope.

The behavioural sciences are sympathetic to covert processes, but only those which are easily measurable, particularly the indices of physiological events. The behaviourists' search for credibility via a psychophysiological path, in the absence of a model by which to discriminate between discreet qualities of consciousness, has resulted in serious anomalies. For example, the concept of 'physiological anxiety' is not a unitary one; criteria assumed to be objective manifestations of anxiety do not match one another and exhibit much less synchronicity than was initially assumed. Significantly, subjective measures of anxiety do not correlate well with physiological measures. This casts doubt on the validity of these so-called 'objective' criteria of subjective processes. It also raises the fundamental question of whether we can meaningfully categorise a broad spectrum of distressing subjective experiences under the blanket concept of 'anxiety' without further differentiation.

Throughout this book, we have highlighted potential clinical roles of cognitive psychology and the phenomenological perspective and tried to illustrate how they can co-exist as complimentary modes of enquiry. A model by which the two systems of study can become integrated is not easily delineated, but we have selected specimen areas of psychopathology to illuminate spheres of reciprocal concern. Some readers may be surprised by the frequency with which depersonalisation and other distortions of 'sense-of-self' and 'self-to-world' are cited throughout the text. It is our conviction that altered states of awareness contribute to the rich array of dysfunctional features which characterise neurotic, psychotic and neurological disorders. Deviation from the accustomed amplitude of self-awareness has repercussions on the interpretation of subsequent experience.

We have deliberately omitted a large and bulky review of phenomenology as a school of philosophy, since we are more interested in the applications of principles in the clinical and psychotherapeutic areas. So the following chapters are not intended to form a comprehensive review of philosophical concepts which underlie models of clinical intervention, nor is this book intended to provide a complete account of psychopathological states.

We address the concerns of the clinician. We have selected complaints and symptoms which people bring to the psychiatric clinic or psychotherapist's room, with a view to subjecting these phenomena to finer analysis than is customary. Examples of problems from clinical practice occur throughout the text and we present conflicting data which are associated with them. But not all deviations from normal experience automatically fall within the rubric of psychopathology; for example, some experiences of heightened awareness constitute a qualitative shift of consciousness which is adaptive and contributes to a sense of well-being. Therefore digression from the usual flow of subjective activity is not in itself a good yardstick of poor mental functioning.

The field of psychopathology would benefit from accumulating knowledge about the relationship between positive and negative deviations of consciousness rather than assume that all deviations worthy of study are maladaptive in quality. In considering the topic of change, we have touched on enlightened experiences of raised hedonic tone, experiences which do not usually fall within the rubric of psychological dysfunction. We believe enriched experiences should be examined with the same exactitude as dysfunctional states, since conceptualisation of adaptive experience may influence treatment strategy and hence the goals of therapy.

Acknowledgements

Thanks to the following people who by word or deed contributed to the evolution of the book: Jeanette Ackroyd, Geoffrey Blowers, Dick Hallam, Annette Maillet, Ariel Stravynski.

Chapter 1

A philosophy of self-body and self-world relations

PHENOMENOLOGY AS A MAINSTREAM PHILOSOPHY

Impartial judgement is a much sought-after commodity. However, unbiased observation, free from the obscurities of prejudiced assessment, is surprisingly elusive. This is particularly so in the human sciences. But why do we need to be objective? In order to assess the merits of objectivity, a crucial set of questions needs to be answered, namely: do the observed properties of an entity reveal its true nature? Are there hidden, 'covert', qualities of an entity, which are more important than its overt features in revealing its essence? How do the assumptions which an observer brings to an investigation influence the conclusion?

Historically, there have been two major attempts to answer these questions, represented by the Rationalist and the Empiricist schools of thought. The Rationalist tradition is typified by Descartes and Berkeley, and, arguably, can be traced to Aristotle. A good synopsis of this tradition and its ramifications can be found elsewhere (see, for example, Loeb 1981). It is important for present purposes to state that the Rationalists assume the existence of fundamental properties, common to several entities, in the form of underlying schemata. These fundamental properties are conceptual, underlying a wide range of processes which, once understood, lead to a broad understanding of external reality. Put simply, the Rationalists advocate the view that the demarcation of covert principles is essential in guiding the nature of things, without which the study of phenomena fails to hang together in a cohesive way.

By contrast, the Empirical tradition, represented by the views of Locke and Hume, puts forward the view that there are no fundamental properties which can be applied to a variety of contexts. Each entity to be studied should therefore be treated with a sort of intellectual '*tabula rasa*', unaffected by assumptions formed on the basis of generalisation. In this sense, the Empirical tradition is antagonistic to that of the Rationalists. The former, unlike the latter, oppose the construction of generalised principles which can be universally applied. For the Empiricist, there can be no 'pure reason' which cuts across the boundaries of things to be investigated.

In practice, both these traditions have significant drawbacks. It is extremely difficult for human beings to assess the various aspects of the external world in isolation, without making some sort of link between them. We barely refrain from infusing some sort of assumed explanation into things, which goes beyond the given data, even though the 'explanation' may have no testable basis. Therefore, both the Rationalists and the Empiricists are faced with the likelihood that any evaluation of a given set of data is idiosyncratic and personal, not systematic or objective. The human shortcoming of premature evaluation, unsatisfactorily countered by Rationalism and Empiricism, inspired the evolution of phenomenology as an intellectual discipline. Phenomenology is a philosophy which has concerned itself with how best to describe phenomena in their own terms, without imposing an interpretation which is the product of intellectual bias. In this sense, it is a philosophy of the description of the nature of things.

The beginnings of phenomenology can be traced to Immanuel Kant, who reflected on the manner in which human beings relate to their respective worlds. In his *Critique of Pure Reason* (1781/1965), Kant asserted that, in gaining information about the world, sensory input undergoes an active process of organisation by the individual receiving it. This organisation was considered to be a function intrinsic to conscious processes. Kant introduced the notion that there is no singular objective world, since prior knowledge of the world is unique to each of us and, therefore, representation of it experientially is idiopathic. This view stresses the individual perception of the observer, so that external objects conform to our highly individualised ways of knowing. Kant further proposed that the mind organises sense impressions using twelve fixed general categories of 'understanding'. These categories of understanding precede learning, and indeed, according to Kant, it is only thanks to these categories that the 'rhapsody of perceptions' is gathered into a connected conciousness. We have to understand basic categories such as 'plurality', 'possibility' and 'causality' in order to make any sense at all of events happening around us.

Kant proposed that experience is connected through human understanding. This connectedness springs from the person's need, not from anything intrinsic to the world. According to Kant, this conceptualisation of external things is the vehicle by which each of us becomes acquainted with the world in an individualistic manner, and explains how the same object may have a diversity of meaning across individuals. In psychological terms, we are 'set' to view objects and events in a particular individualistic way, the perceptual set being determined by acquired, motivational factors.

Georg Hege 1 (1807/1929) was impressed by Kant's assertion that each individual's experience of external reality is unique. However, Hegel considered the idea of a fixed set of categories of understanding to be too rigid. Hegel proposed an alternative, but related, view to that of Kant, which was that consciousness is composed of a series of dialectical (bi-polar) constructs, forming the dimensions along which external reality is validated. These dialectical constructs are not fixed or shared across individuals, but are infinite, and they apply not only to perception of a phenomenon but to any subsequent ideas the person may form about its quantitative or qualitative nature. Hegel made the first attempt at unravelling the structure of consciousness. He suggested that we formulate general categories of understanding by discovering the bi-polar dialectic of appearances. He proposed that, by making a synthesis of the two poles, the bi-polar construct can be transcended by a meta-category. For example, 'red' and 'blue' would form a dialectic transcended by the synthesis category 'colour'; for something to be described as 'rational', there must be some conception of 'irrational', transcended by the synthesis category 'logic'. In this way, apparent contradictions in our thoughts and perceptions are made compatible with each other by forming a larger concept that transcends and synthesises the original two poles. Thus, two events or objects which are evaluated as different, by virtue of occupying contrary positions within a specific dialectic can be incorporated into the overall meaning structure, by virtue of their conceptual relatedness. Hegel construed the history of human ideas as progressing in a dialectical fashion, in such a way that new data lead to modification and expansion of categories and meta-categories.

Hegel's idea of the dialectic was abstract and limited to how ideas about the world are formed but his dialectic was applied in more concrete form by Karl Marx to the concept of social development. Marx (1867/1967) used Hegel's philosophy of dialectics in proposing that society itself progresses through dialectical stages representing bi-polar categories of social consciousness, which are eventually transcended by a unifying higher consciousness. The two polar opposites of bourgeoisie and working class can be transcended by 'society'. Social structure can be reconceptualised in terms of a unifying classless socialism. Marx termed this synthesis 'dialectic materialism'. Of more relevance to us here is the idea that the organisation of consciousness takes on a bi-polar structure, which patterns our evaluation of the world. The same notion is utilised today and forms the basis of certain self-report measurement techniques, such as Osgood's (1971) semantic differential and Kelly's (1955) constructs. One of Hegel's more profound syntheses was the assimilation of thought and feeling into 'existence'. Hegel viewed existence as a more fundamental unit of consciousness than either thought or feeling. In other words, both thought and feeling reflect distinct aspects of a person's existence and at an existential level, reflected by the experience of being, neither emotion nor cognition are singly of greater importance.

Kierkegaard (1844/1957) took up Hegel's concept of existence as the fundamental unit of personal knowledge and suggested that a core process, vital to each individual, is the development of self-awareness. An important aspect of self-awareness is the appreciation of choice which an individual commands. The realisation that the current mode of existence is not inevitable, but is self-determined, is for Kierkegaard a fundamental personal responsibility. This notion of awareness of existence is for Kierkegaard a moral issue, whereby the individual has the option to be aware or not. He explored the dilemma of choice in publications such as *Either/Or* (1843/1954), in which the reader is encouraged to confront the personal responsibility for existence through facing a series of difficult moral choices. The dilemma of self-awareness gives rise to the experience of 'dread', an emotion which is generated by the alarming realisation that the nature of selfhood is not predetermined but open to infinite transformation. Kierkegaard's perspective gave rise to *'existenz-analyse'* or existentialism. *Existenz-analyse* reflects the uniqueness of core experience and stresses the importance of self-awareness for each individual, as a duty of being in the world. In doing so, existentialism reflects a value system, which has become an important aspect of contemporary ethical philosophy.

The progression of thinking from Kant to Kierkegaard produced a growth in interest in the individual psyche. Today, the significance of this development may be difficult for us fully to comprehend, since in modern contemporary life, individual psychology is taken for granted and is part of our conceptual thinking. Nowadays, for example, it may seem obvious that our appreciation of the external world and our construing of reality varies across individuals. However, prior to Kant, external reality was considered to be reciprocated by the respective experiences it produced. Nowadays, there is a greater awareness that this is not the case and that distal stimuli are reconstructed in a manner unique to each individual. An implication of idiopathic percepts is that there is some form of intervening variable, lying between the external world and the way each individual makes sense of it. Strictly speaking, we cannot talk of shared perceptual experience, in that every individual will carry a unique sense of being-in-the-world. In the face of the same external event, its appraisal will be constructed by and therefore unique to its beholder.

At the same time as Kierkegaard was defining *existenz-analyse*, Hegel's synthesis of thought and feeling into 'existence' had different repercussions in academic circles. German-speaking academics were beginning to focus on how existence, as 'being in the here and now', could be demarcated. They were interested in treating 'being' as a measurable entity. More specifically, Hegel inspired later attempts to understand experience as a series of fleeting units of sensation, each temporal 'unit of being' amounting to a sample of the overall sensation of awareness. Being was viewed as a continuous process, a sample of the here and now representing a snapshot of the more global mechanics of existence.

Working from the premise that personal sensory impressions possess a highly individualised style, Franz Brentano guided scientific psychological investigation away from the positivist tradition espoused by Comte and Wundt. The problem he addressed was as follows: how can the concept of personalised and idiopathic experience be subjected to empirical rather than philosophical enquiry? Brentano (1874/1973) argued that description was the key to capturing experience and so description should be the first aim of psychology. A phenomenon should be understood in its natural context before a causal explanation is imposed upon it. He differentiated between what he termed 'genetic' and 'descriptive' psychology. The 'genetic' or exploratory part of psychology should come only after description. All aspects of a phenomenon should be considered relevant and not ordered prior to observation. This approach contrasted with the positivist approach, in which experience was, and still is, construed as bound to hypothetical systems beyond lived experience.

Brentano refused to step beyond experience in order to explain experiential phenomena. Accurate description of consciousness was viewed as the precursor of all other knowledge, since in the final analysis all knowledge is subjective. By contrast, the positivist school regarded an interest in introspective experience as a self-indulgent activity, anecdotal and prone to arbitrary bias. The task of positivist science in psychology was to go beyond the limitations of potential observer bias and progress towards absolute laws of truth which are irrefutable. In order to do this, positivists have chosen to study material which is essentially objective in criteria and measurability. For example, the positivist approach to the measurement of subjective sensation is exemplified by the use of externally validated self-report data and mapping these through objective mathematical power functions, e.g. Stevens's (1961) work on psychophysics.

The history of psychological positivism illustrates a tendency to fragment experience into levels. For example, in experimental psychology, assumptions are made that a person processes a stimulus at physical and semantic levels separately, since such separate processing seems logical to the experimenter. Within the field of medicine, the development of neurological science has persuaded many intellectuals that physical entities such as brain tissue and neurotransmitters are somehow 'fundamental' to the psyche. The notion that experience is *caused* by organic material events is opposed in phenomenological thinking; for the phenomenologists, the subjective and biological components of positivist systems are incompatible – the physical and the subjective do not directly influence each other. Experience is not given from a physical source, but from processes contained within the psyche. This position means that though the experiential and biological realms are both implicated in self-hood, only experiential factors are directly related to subjective space. Indeed, for phenomenologists, physical and psychic entities are incomparable and outside of one another's spheres of influence. This is a fundamental premise of phenomenology, with important implications for methodology. We will return to these methodological issues at several points throughout the text.

One of Brentano's concerns was the human shortcoming of forming premature affiliation with explanatory concepts. He viewed human nature as a liability in forming causal hypotheses and seeking plausible confirmation prior to the variables involved being fully known. One outcome arising out of this shortcoming is that variables become falsely implicated as a causal process of an event before the event itself has become exposed and laid before the investigator. Without knowing the full nature of the dependent variable, its corresponding independent variables are impossible to tease out.

Edmund Husserl was a distinguished student of Brentano who attempted to give a more systematic form to some of Brentano's reflections on science and description. Husserl became preoccupied with what he termed the 'crisis of science', brought about through a readiness of scientific thinkers to adopt assumptions ostensibly arrived at by common sense, but which in actuality bore no resemblance to the true nature of the object of study. Husserl (1970a) coined the phrase 'the natural attitude' to refer to schema fraught with logical error due to a failure to distinguish between metaphor, description and explanation. He emphasised the view that as human beings we have an unfortunate tendency to attribute explanation to all things we observe, and that attempts at explanation are an obstacle to our attempts at evaluation of the thing itself. This apparent weakness in human functioning, the tendency to adopt attributional styles of reasoning, may have survival value within an everyday life ecological context, where the rapid formulation of hypotheses may be required concerning the nature of the physical and social environment, followed by instantaneous acceptance or rejection of such hypotheses in order to effect action. However, this 'magnetism of explanation', as Heider (1958) later called it, is vehemently suspended in phenomenological circles in order to enhance the collection of data pertaining to the natural characteristics of things, rather than premature speculation concerning their causation.

According to Husserl, we are only correct to enquire into the relations between instantaneous variables, rather than those coming before or after an observation. Husserl termed this approach 'eidetic reduction'. Eidetic reduction is the examination of intervariable relations existing only at the time of the observed event, and these relations only have meaning if related to the subject's consciousness of the event. Because consciousness is always actively directed towards something, Husserl termed it *intentional*; intentional not in the sense of directly intended, but in the sense that there is always a purposeful background theme which connects the elements of conscious awareness. Husserl and Brentano introduced this actively directed consciousness of the observer as the background which illuminates and gives sense to what is perceived in the field of observation. We capture this subjective background, or eidetic context, by focusing on the content of perception, particularly how a percept appears to the subject, revealing how sense has been made of the percept.

For Husserl, the first major task of phenomenology was to bracket out everyday assumptions and deal only with the data available; we are only correct to enquire into the relations of instantaneous variables, not those ordered temporally – these are things seen in their 'essence'. For Husserl, the starting point of any investigation is this psychological stripping away of the everyday associations surrounding a phenomenon to reveal the phenomenon as a unit by itself. He suggested, following Brentano, that this could be done by treating both the experience and the phenomenon experienced as a single unit or 'act'. When a subject views an object or an event, the characteristics of what the subject sees are not only defined by the object but by the subject's predominant expectancies. The observed is therefore always a product of the consciousness that is observing.

Post-war phenomenologists such as Sartre (1957) and Merleau-Ponty (1965) reflected upon the role of consciousness. For them both, all mental operations (thoughts, perceptions, verbal and nonverbal processing, psychic and somatic events) in consciousness need to be considered as equally important constituents, with no priorities accorded to any element. Sartre, in particular, insisted that consciousness includes several layers of self-reflection and that whatever one is conscious of is related to what one is not conscious of, and that we have the additional ability to be conscious of our consciousness. Sartre's theory of emotion is of some interest, since it predates the approach of recent motor theorists who view emotional experience and muscular activity as part of the same action system. Sartre considered emotion a product of the frustrated ability to transform and act on the world instrumentally. Hence, emotion is for Sartre a 'magical incantation'. The physiology of emotion results from a symbolic struggle to do more than is possible when nothing is possible. Sartre's theory was an advance over the then contemporary notions of emotion as a kind of surplus energy, and the conative aspects of Sartre's theory of emotion as directed intentions are not dissimilar from current cognitive theories (see Denzin 1984).

PHENOMENOLOGY IN THE MENTAL HEALTH CONTEXT

Existentialism

Martin Heidegger was Husserl's assistant but disagreed with Husserl's emphasis on searching for the essences of objects and acts. Heidegger argued that instead of trying to reduce events to their essence and strip away the context, we are better off trying to find true meaning in the context of the immediate concerns of the person's existence. Heidegger therefore grounded consciousness in the concerns of everyday life. He called his major work *Sein und Zeit*, which is usually translated as *Being and Time* (1927) but might more aptly be termed 'being in the here and now'. He stated that all efforts of the existential analytic have one goal: to find a means of investigating the meaning of being. He linked this search for meaning with mental health, proposing that lack of meaning was a core feature of psychopathological states.

Heidegger's approach to experience was from the analysis of what is portrayed at any given moment in time, or *'Dasein-analysis'* ('existence-analysis'). Heidegger gave primacy to mood as the main clue to unravelling a person's existential concerns. He stated that the world is pre-given precisely as felt-meaning, and that the grounding consciousness of the world is primordial affect. According to Heidegger, mood is the sheer sense of how a person stands in relation to the world. Mood is here-and-now attunement and predates any cognitive interpretations. In particular, he described the state of 'dread' as a profound alienation from the stream of everyday life. This alienated state, in which everyday engagement is diminished, was for Heidegger a state in which the individual is confronted by the structure of *Dasein* and its subjective and acausal nature. Contemporary psychiatrists of the day, for example, Ludwig Binswanger, used Heidegger's analysis of dread as a way of understanding psychopathology, particularly in attempting to describe disturbances of emotion.

The idea of applying *Dasein-analysis* to a discrete sample of consciousness attracted considerable interest. Binswanger, Boss, Minkowski, Straus, von Gebsattel and Frankl formed the first wave of existential psychiatrists to apply Heidegger's 'Analytic of Existence' to mental illness. Frankl (1952) invented his own form of therapy called 'Logotherapy', which he developed while in a concentration camp and which he based on the premise that it is essential for survival to have a goal. The idea that life goals are important to health and well-being figures prominently in the modern existential conceptualisation of self-actualisation (Maslow 1968) and features in current concepts of cognitive psychopathology (e.g. Stein and Trabasso 1992). Existential psychiatrists were more specific than Heidegger in their application of *Dasein* to problem areas. They attempted to understand the meaning of specific psychiatric symptoms in existential terms. Straus, for example, discusses the idea that hallucinations originate in distorted sense modalities. But this input distortion has no ready and meaningful interpretation to match up with it, so one is invented, seen or heard (Straus 1966: 287), and this produces a pathological mode of being-in-the-world. It is interesting to compare this *Existenz*-analysis of hallucinations with more recent cognitive experiments showing how under conditions of ambiguity (e.g. white noise) subjects are more likely to see or hear patterns conforming to pre-existing meaning structures (Jakes and Hemsley 1986).

An important contribution of this group was to advocate that experiences generally considered physiological or biological in origin could only be understood in terms of the emotional meaning matrix of the person's current state of being-in-the-world. Ludwig Binswanger wrote that

> Heidegger . . . affords empirical psychopathological research, a new methodological and material basis that goes beyond its previous scientific framework and gives a key by means of which the psychiatrist can ascertain and describe the phenomena he investigates in their full phenomenal content and intrinsic context.
>
> (Binswanger 1963: 202)

This brought them into conflict with more accepted clinical practice, in that the traditional approach at that time was to search for specific underlying (organic or psychodynamic) causes for psychiatric symptoms. For Binswanger, the basic constituent of *Dasein-analysis* was an individual's experience of being-in-an-event; understanding of the world is achieved through constructed interpretation, a subjective context which Binswanger termed the 'meaning-matrix'.

Binswanger exemplifies clinical phenomenology in his objection to the assumption that a mentally ill human being is a 'sick organism' exhibiting signs of some underlying biological disorder. He rejected the belief that anatomy is the seat of psychological dysfunction. The existentialists viewed the physical being as conceptually unrelated to the unique schemata constructed in conscious life. Coupled with this was the notion that the understanding of an individual's present behaviour is only achievable through consideration of his present being-in-the-world in its entirety. On this basis, he found organic psychiatry to have an irrelevant focus.

Binswanger also isolated himself from psychoanalysis. Freud stated that the concept of unconscious processes is a necessary one because 'the data of consciousness are exceedingly defective' (Freud 1957: 64). Phenomenologists took exception to this view, since it was interpreted as negating the importance of conscious experience. They interpreted the psychoanalysts' methodology as an obstinate resistance to take 'what is experienced' seriously; the effect of Freudian theory was seen as the relegation of consciousness to the role of 'symbolisation' of other (i.e. unconscious) material. The psychoanalytic preoccupation with unconscious processes shifted attention away from existence in its immediate form, a diversion which prompted much antagonism from phenomenology. Binswanger (1963) commented that for the psychoanalyst to talk of conscious experience as a symbolic expression of some deeper unconscious element is to attempt the removal of consciousness from the field of investigation altogether. For the existentialist, an intrapsychic sign is an impossibility. That is, one cannot experience something as a sign of an inner state or emotion. At best, one can experience a feeling or image that may be said to represent a wider feeling, but this does not detract from the value of the present (conscious) feeling as a significant entity in itself.

Binswanger postulated that one of the implications of the psychoanalytic method in adopting the notion of unconscious 'causes' of experience is that experience is split off from meaningful motivation. By employing intrapsychic symbolism, the psychoanalyst conceives of the meaning of a behaviour occurring subsequent to its motivation. According to the psychoanalytic model, an aberrant behaviour may be precipitated by an unconscious desire; the desire is then given a facile meaning by the beholder, which is conceptually compatible with his or her current conscious plans but does not reveal the true motivation. However, the phenomenologist limits her/himself to present consciousness, so that motivation and meaning are inextricably interwoven. Binswanger writes:

> Unconscious desire is the vehicle whereby meaning and explanation in psychoanalysis are derived; in dream image analysis, where a knife is said to 'mean' a phallus, or a suitcase a vulva, understanding falls short of the patient if it is not further asked what the phallus or vulva means to the individual. But the full phenomenal value of the knife in the world of the patient must be 'laid forth' before the analysist can understand what phallus means to the patient. The conclusion that knife means phallus, presupposes that all meaning-direction emanates from a biological need. This ignores the possibility that these biological needs are themselves enmeshed in a larger meaning matrix. The full meaning of the symbol is thus attenuated a priori in psychoanalysis by limiting its context to only one aspect of the patient's world.
>
> (Binswanger 1963: 253).

Ironically, the objectives and methods of therapy for the early phenomenological therapists were obscured by the fact that the early wave of existentialists were unaware of their own inability to escape the pervasive influence of psychoanalysis. Binswanger himself showed a straying of principles into the analytic model, and there is little effort by him to transcend his own medical and interpretative role in his clinical case histories. Nonetheless, there was a general disquiet over the psychoanalysts' emphasis on libidinal conflict, and this disquiet partly came from outside of clinical circles. Sartre (1957), though not himself a psychopathologist, expressed his doubts that the volitional component of human nature is based on libidinal energy. He felt that psychoanalysis should be much broader in its conception of the prime motivational dynamic, preferring something akin to a drive-to-be as a volition to obtain or reject full awareness of individual existence. The phenomenologists' negative identification with formal psychoanalysis and medicine was to set the major parameters of clinical phenomenology in the context of modern psychopathology.

Client-centred psychology

On the other side of the Atlantic, the concept of the 'phenomenal self' seeped into the literature, reflecting the aspiration of understanding personal psychological events on the subject's own terms, i.e. an understanding from the point of reference of the beholder. This aspiration was adopted by theoretical psychotherapists of the humanist tradition.

The idea of measuring personal meaning in terms of a bi-polar dialectic also became fashionable. The personal construct psychology of Kelly (1955) was extremely influential in providing subjective philosophy with a psychological vocabulary. Kelly spoke of the way in which we evaluate the world, through our structured perception of it, which is moulded by experience. Kelly proposed that our evaluative perception is organised along bi-polar dimensions, which he termed 'constructs'. The 'Kelly's Grid' technique of clinical assessment has evolved out of this dialectic approach. Grid techniques involve establishing how highly personalised dimensions of evaluation interrelate in the context of elements (in the therapy context, elements usually consist of significant people in the subject's life). This clinical procedure charts out how a variety of personally-important criteria by which the subject assesses the world mesh together, giving some insight into the subject's world-view. Conveniently, a grid analysis can be presented in two-dimensional form as a matrix of appraisals. A major value of the technique lies in its ability to reveal how construct criteria normally used in assessing a restricted set of elements are applied by the subject to elements for which the construct is normally latent, or ostensibly does not form part of conscious judgement.

Osgood *et al.*'s semantic differential consists of a series of scales stretched between two antonymous adjectives and divided into a number of steps, usually seven. Osgood *et al.* (1971) adopts a three-dimensional space to describe ratings according to an evaluation (good–bad) axis, a potency (strong–weak) axis and an activity (active–passive) axis.

Kelly's (1955) grid method seems to offer advantages over Osgood *et al.*'s differential in accounting for the hierarchial nature of personal evaluation. The grid operates at the two levels of elements and constructs and establishes a flexible 'reality reference space' for the client, which can be applied to a number of activities and complex behaviours. But this grid is always based on the client's meaning system, not prescribed by the experimenter's understanding.

The repertory grid provides a means of assessing relations between a subject's constructs and the world informed by them. Personal construct theory guides the clinician's examination of the patient's discourse at the moment of its generation, while the grid provides an account of the relations between its parts and significant features of the patient's universe *a posteriori*. This divergence between the spontaneous account and the need to quantify it places some limits on the descriptions offered by the patient but this should not be seen as unnecessarily restrictive. Even in open conversation, sentences often express a speaker's ideas in shorthand form. Several points may be condensed within a single phrase which seems obscure; alternatively, an excess of words may carry only a single idea. The art of the clinician is to tease out the ideas the patient expresses in terms of singular dimensions of construct-contrast form, as Kelly suggests, confirming the patient's meaning by feeding back his or her understanding of what the patient means and obtaining clarification by confirmation or amendment.

Kelly emphasised the uniqueness of constructs to each person, and demonstrated with examples how individuals often use them in highly idiosyncratic ways. These demonstrations are the greatest proof that one cannot treat too lightly the words of another; nor should one assume that just because two people speak a 'common language' that their shared words mean the same things for each of them.

Around the same time, Carl Rogers, whose primary interest was the 'here-and-now' processes active in psychotherapy, was developing his client-centred approach (Rogers 1951). Rogers saw the essential ingredient of personal change as being self-understanding and self-acceptance. He took the view that human beings are inherently problem-solving animals who constantly strive to make sense of the world through a progressively more accurate interpretation of internal and external events. He asserted that constructive investigation of the client's 'phenomenological field' should be attempted, with a view to fostering a re-evaluation by the client of him/herself, particularly in relation to others. Rogers upheld an idealistic goal for the therapist, namely, the acquisition of a full understanding of the client's perceptual-evaluative field. It is this core understanding of the client's inner world, in the here and now, which Rogers referred to as 'empathy'. To facilitate this process, Rogers (1961) developed the procedure of non-directive counselling. This is a formal clinical method, which is used by a great many modern-day clinicians and therapists.

Rogerian counselling has its pragmatic application within the dialogue between client and therapist and is a means of establishing and maintaining rapport. The client is encouraged to talk through the presenting problem in an unrestrained way, while the therapist interjects from time to time in order to reflect back what has been said, usually in paraphrased form. This reflective process serves to clarify points which the client has made and to act as a prompt to further introspection and self-reflection. The therapist avoids asking leading questions and in doing so avoids imposing his or her own structure on the client's problem. An important process variable of therapy was the client's increased awareness in the evaluation of self and world; the gaining of insight through making explicit what before was implicit assumption.

Many therapists keen to approach clinical problems from a phenomenological perspective avoided becoming embedded in theoretical debate, and were instead anxious to experiment with ways of, in R. D. Laing's phrase, 'going directly to the patients themselves and keeping to a minimum the discussion of the historical, theoretical, and practical issues raised particularly *vis-à-vis* psychiatry and psycho-analysis' (Laing 1965: 16). Rogerian counselling serves to promote a broader view by providing an optimal interpersonal environment in which the client's thoughts about self and world can develop to a meaningful level. For Rogers, this involved the client making a clearer differentiation between self-experience and the outside world (Rogers 1951). Rogers rejected psychoanalytic notions of the unconscious, replacing it with the concept of the preconscious. The preconscious comprises data not currently lying within the centre of consciousness, but which is nonetheless potentially accessible to awareness (and self-modification) given optimum conditions.

It appears that Rogers was not particularly interested in the phenomenological movement in Europe, but, interestingly, at Rice University in 1964 he spoke as the advocate of phenomenology, suggesting the approach might be a powerful alternative to behaviourism and psychoanalysis. The complex and subtle relationship between Rogers and the phenomenological movement is outlined by Spiegelberg (1972). Suffice it to say here that in later work (e.g. Rogers 1976) there is considerable identification in retrospect with the phenomenological movement, particularly the Husserlian notion of consciousness as consciousness-of-something, that is, consciousness with reference to the construing of self and external world, as embraced within Husserl's concept of 'intentionality' in perceptual processes. The factor these writers had in common was the shared target of enquiry, that is, the client's orientation to the experiential framework.

Subsequent practitioners have been influenced to some degree by the client-centred approach, since the approach represented a fundamental shift in clinical procedure. In the USA, Beck (1976) acknowledged Rogers's emphasis on a warm, genuine and empathic therapeutic atmosphere and upheld the aim of 'working with the patient as collaborator'. Though Beck felt that client-centred techniques could be refined and developed, he gave the Rogerian approach guarded support: 'Only a few popular therapies on the current scene meet the minimal requirements for a system of psychotherapy. Rogerian, or client-centred, therapy is reasonably specific in its prescribed procedures but explicitly avoids a comprehensive model of psychopathology' (Beck 1976: 309). Beck (1976) set out a series of ground rules for evaluating systems of psychotherapy and suggested that psychotherapeutic models of good quality should exhibit the following characteristics: the approach should be outlined with sufficient clarity as to be replicable, while at the same time allowing flexibility between therapists; the efficacy of the intervention strategy should have empirical support, and improvement should be sustained at long-term follow-up; there should be well-validated reasons for focusing on specific aspects of the patient's problem; and the process of change should be attributable to particular stages of the treatment procedure by longitudinal assessment at successive intervals throughout the intervention.

Jaspers's clinical phenomenology

Whilst some phenomenologists, such as Straus (1966) and Frankl (1952), related psychiatric problems to the motivation to make sense of existence, a strong tradition had already become established in nineteenth century Europe by Bretano and Husserl which aimed to describe features of the mental state, irrespective of how they were generated. During the twentieth century, much of the drive to remain with the here-and-now experience of psychological dysfunction is attributed to psychiatrist and philosopher Karl Jaspers. Spiegelberg (1972), in his noted work on the history of phenomenology in psychology and psychiatry, credits Jaspers as the major initiator of phenomenological thinking in psychopathology. The influences that have shaped the views of a given individual are often implicit or become obscured through history. Jaspers is no exception. Though Jaspers acknowledged the work of Husserl, he stated that his own work would have taken the same course even had Husserl been unknown to him. It is a matter of debate to what degree Jaspers was influenced by Brentano and Husserl, since applying the principle of the 'bracketing out' of assumptions in descriptive psychology is valued by all three.

In 1913, Jaspers published his first edition of *Allgemeine Psychopathologie* (General Psychopathology), a work which was elaborated over several further editions, culminating in an edition which was translated into English by Hamilton and Hoenig in 1963. This work was the cornerstone of descriptive psychopathology throughout the first half of the twentieth century and has been the inspiration behind shorter works, including Fish's *Clinical Psychopathology* (1967) and *Symptoms in the Mind* (Sims 1988). A common feature of all three works is the structuring of the text in terms of subjective features rather than in terms of psychiatric diagnoses, these features serving to give a different order to clinical evaluation. For example, all three authors structure their texts according to the perspectives of self-awareness, style of self-report and perceptual processes rather than by diagnostic grouping. In the process, the reader is furnished with a great deal of discussion concerning the subjective meaning which underlies overt signs and symptoms. In doing so, these writers have added a great deal to the current knowledge of dysfunctional psychological states, particularly the psychoses. The hallmark of descriptive phenomenology is that the clinical description offered contains a critical awareness of the perspective from which it was described, a point which distinguishes disciplined from anecdotal phenomenological studies (De Koning and Jenner 1982).

Most phenomenological psychiatrists utilise a diagnostic framework and regard the major diagnostic systems as possessing some pragmatic value, especially the

World Health Organisation system (ICD 10) and the American Psychiatric Association system (DSM-III-R). However, the clinical phenomenologist is not content with merely a diagnosis. As Sims puts it, 'It is important to try to reach the patient's subjective meaning and not just be satisfied that the response is abnormal' (Sims 1988: 9). Jaspers (1963) distinguishes between experiences with which the clinician can empathise, and features which are 'un-understandable'. The concept of un-understandability is important, since it essentially refers to experiences which are of a psychotic nature and which, according to Jaspers, do not arise from any source discernible to the observer. Such experiences are therefore beyond the scope of empathic understanding. Jaspers's view has helped clarify the distinction between overvalued ideas, i.e. over-emphasised ideation with which the subject is preoccupied and in which an inappropriate level of affective response is invested, and delusions, which Jaspers viewed as arising out of a radical transformation of meaning. During the transformation from non-deluded to delusional thinking, a special sense of awareness occurs in which mundane stimuli are imbued with new meaning and significance. The patient is immersed within a qualitatively distinct subjective atmosphere as the delusion is hatched. This changed quality of subjective experience is considered by Jaspers to be beyond the bounds of understanding, in empathic terms, and is meaningful to no one but the beholder.

Jaspers's intention in writing *General Psychopathology* was to provide an overview of psychopathology in terms of conscious subjective events. Perhaps more importantly, Jaspers outlined the principles by which the task should be fulfilled. Like Binswanger, with whom he exchanged correspondence, Jaspers rejected both psychoanalysis and neurology as routes to understanding, dismissing them both as 'mythological' bases from which the exploration of consciousness was doomed to failure. Jaspers did not set out to provide a philosophy of existence, as, for example, Heidegger had done. Instead, Jaspers set out to describe both the psychic life of individuals exhibiting psychopathology, and the methods by which the psyche could be investigated, through interaction with his patients. He took a great deal of care in recording personalised accounts of abnormal experiences, both at their time of occurrence and through patients' lucid retrospective descriptions. Jaspers found that the prevailing literary accounts of dysfunctional experience were inadequate, since they bore little resemblance to the experiences his patients described. As a result, he began to construct his own psychological model of consciousness, which encompassed both normal and abnormal experience. As Spiegelberg points out, the phenomenological psychopathologists have invaded the field of phenomenological psychology to such an extent that they no longer distinguish between psychology and psychopathology. Most of these psychopathologists clearly felt that they had to build their own psychology.

Jaspers was concerned to develop a phenomenological method which added structure to investigative methods, and was therefore keen to do more than simply accumulate an endless series of clinical data. He was dubious about the popularity of empirical research in academic circles, and felt that the reporting of statistical relationships between variables was of little value without reference to the data's significance to an overall research perspective. Jaspers was concerned that the presentation of empirical data was becoming fashionable to such an extent that mathematical and statistical presentation seemed sufficient justification for the research itself. This was an unacceptable state of affairs to Jaspers, who felt that the core purpose of psychological investigation was taking second place to the accumulation of numerically compatible criteria. He reflected:

> Salvation is thought to lie in experiments where results are either expressed in figures or are objectively demonstrated or plotted as a curve. The upholders of such views are guilty of one omission. They fail to train themselves in psychological methods and therefore may be charged with uncritical thinking. Observation is not enough. If we are to obtain some clear, communicable concepts and if we are to reach an adequate differentiation of our field, valid thinking in addition is essential, otherwise no advance in our knowledge will take place.
>
> (Jaspers 1963: 4).

Jaspers saw the need to develop a meaningful structure by which psychological investigations could be systemised, so that the full implications of the relationship between two statistically-related variables could be assessed. Such a view is consistent with that of Wittgenstein (1953), who expressed the view that human behaviour is on the whole insufficiently understood in that there is a tendency for theoreticians in the human sciences to feel satisfied that behaviour has been 'explained' if its antecedents have been identified. For Wittgenstein, the identification of an event contiguous with a behaviour merely suggests the event is somehow potentially implicated as an antecedent of that behaviour. This provides no measure of understanding of how the antecedent and its consequence are causally linked. Jaspers was concerned to fill this gap, by determining the meaningful connectedness between particular symptoms or bizarre behaviours and the subjective activity around which the phenomena arose.

Jaspers distinguished between two senses of the term 'understanding', namely, static understanding and genetic understanding. The distinction reflects two lines of enquiry: static understanding is achieved through the analysis of experience at a given moment in time. For example, static understanding is achieved by forming a picture of what the subject is experiencing in the here and now, irrespective of what has occurred prior to the experience or what occurs subsequently. This corresponds to the concept of *Dasein-analysis*, discussed previously. Genetic understanding, on the other hand, refers to an appreciation of how the components of awareness become crystallised into 'experience' through study of the relatedness of subjective events in which experience has arisen. Genetic understanding is therefore concerned with the process by which an experience has come about, and is achieved through examining the subjective meaning of events which have resulted in the experience or behaviour under consideration.

Jaspers was interested in both the form and content of experience. The content of experience comprises the perceptual and evaluative processes, the concerns of the subject. In the psychiatric context, content reflects the preoccupations described by the person, including the source to which the subject attributes them. Content reflects the thoughts and percepts as they are presented, and content exposes the meaning-matrix of the person. For example, an individual may be immersed in the conviction of being the victim of persecution and may be fearful and in search of protection. The form of experience, on the other hand, is a product of the observer's abstraction, a clinical reconceptualisation of the significance of the experiential phenomena. The form of experience is a reconceptualisation of the patient's presentation, so that analysis takes place outside of the parameters of the patient's self-report. Detached from the patient's volition, the clinician may judge the patient's conviction to exhibit a *paranoid* flavour, and to be *false* and *unshakeable*. The viewpoint is constructed from a position apart from that of the beholder of the belief. Form is therefore a deduction. The form is never referred to directly by the patient, since the patient is interested only in the content of the distress, usually with much attention to attribution (for a further discussion of form and content, see, for example, Sims 1988: 12–13).

Jaspers created a framework which forms a systematic observational method by which the various lines of enquiry can be contextualised with regard to their meaning and possible significance. He objected to theory-driven deductive reasoning because of its narrowness, arguing that investigative methods should be task-oriented, not theoretically determined. To that end, he believed passionately that the organisation of investigative objectives should be born out of the minutiae of detailed description, rather than arise out of abstract philosophical notions marked by their obliqueness and irrelevance to his patients' subjective characteristics. His position is exemplified in the following statement:

> There have been periods in which great value has been placed on speculative and deductive thinking, based on principles that sought to comprehend and explain everything without the test of experience. Such thinking was more highly valued then than the irksome examination of particulars. These were periods in which philosophy tried to create from 'above' what only experience could bring from 'below'.

Predictably, he added:

> Our rejection of purely deductive and barren philosophical theorising is justified but it is often linked regrettably with the opposite misconception, that the only useful approach is to go on with the collection of particular experiences. It is thought better to amass data blindly than sit down and think. From this follows a contempt for the activity of thinking, which alone gives a place to facts, a plan to work to, a standpoint for observation and the passionate drive for rewarding scientific goals.

> Jaspers (1963: 16)

It is sometimes argued that assessment of the subjective world of another human being can never be objective, because either the classification system or the act of classification is the product of the subjectivity of others. Whenever a judgement is made it is inevitably subjective, since it is formed entirely within the perceptual structure of the observer. This is a major problem for phenomenologists, since all concepts have utility and reflect the intentionality of the observer.

Spiegelberg (1975) is less optimistic than Husserl in the achievement of objective purity of description, even when descriptive terms are devoid of premature explanatory concepts. This is because the observer, at the outset of the enquiry, inevitably comes to the situation accompanied by preconceived ideas and a preformed perceptual style. Thus, previous knowledge and experience impose a predetermined organisation or gestalt upon the configuration of data. According to Spiegelberg, the best we can aspire to is the articulation of these preconceived notions. For Jaspers, the preconceived notions are revealed by the lines of enquiry which the clinician adopts, and since these are always influenced by existing presupposition, at best one can only specify them.

Jaspers's emphasis on critique and revision of methodology inevitably begs justification of the fundamental model which underlies his own reconstruction of the structure of experience. The full relatedness (and therefore the distinction) between processes such as 'attention', 'emotion', 'awareness', 'perception' and 'feeling' are as yet poorly defined and not thoroughly self-evident. We do not know to what degree even the basic phenomenological constructs of consciousness are valid as the core material of 'being'. Concepts undergo continuous transformation over time and their value lies in their function to elucidate. Within the framework of knowledge, all concepts undergo critical review and, ironically, serve to organise information which eventually results in their self-destruction. As Heidegger (1927) wrote:

> The real movement of the sciences takes place when their basic concepts undergo a more or less radical revision which is transparent to itself. The level which a science has reached is determined by how far it is capable of a crisis in its basic concepts. In such immanent crises the very relationship between positive investigative inquiry and those things themselves that are under interrogation comes to a point where it begins to totter.
>
> (Heidegger 1927: 29)

Perhaps Jaspers's lasting value, of which he would be proud, is the provision of a clear investigative structural method, upon which efforts to refine an investigative model can be focused.

COMPUTER ANALOGUE MODELS AND THE PROBLEM OF MEANING

It can be argued that attempts to apply the phenomenological method belong mainly to the domain of the social sciences, in particular, sociology and linguistics. The reason for this is that the concepts applied in the study of social reflections and verbal reasoning recognise the contribution of self-as-actor in constructing social reality. In tandem, the constructionist orientation of cognitive psychology has helped cast a new light on aberrant thoughts and actions. Conversely cognitive science, as the technology of information processing, has tended by virtue of its experimental nature to be modular, laboratory-based and hypothetico-deductive. Often, cognitive science has used computer analogue models to understand how memory modules or semantic-processing modules function, albeit often in isolation.

The source of inspiration of cognitive science for most of this present century has not been psychology, but communications science (for example, the filter models of information processing developed in the 1950s along with the advent of the signal and information technology of RC filters and transistor networks have been highly influential in shaping the focus of investigation). Ideas borrowed from computer science provided concepts such as the soft-wired and hard-wired operations of the central nervous system, drawing a distinction between the innate pre-programmed subjective responses common to all human beings, and those which are determined by learning and experience. Recently, concepts such as connectionism, parallel-distributed processing and chaos theory have been adopted by cognitive scientists as a means of furthering understanding of human psychological functioning. Analogies drawn between the brain and available communications models lead to assumptions about the connections of input and output, levels of processing the stages of perception and action, and the role of internal representations of stimuli. These connecting stages are hypothetical, incorporating abstract levels of description by what Kluger and Turvey (1987) termed 'boxology', i.e. black boxes depicting hypothetical rather than actual processes. Arguably, the black box is getting smaller, the more that the properties of human experiential functions are investigated.

Many clinical observations fail to validate computer analogue models, and defy a strict division of events into thought and feeling, perception and action, physical and mental responses. Richard Williams (1987) has recently addressed some of these concerns in an article entitled 'Can cognitive psychology offer a meaningful account of meaningful human action?' He makes the point that meaningfulness as a human possibility fits awkwardly into a model of logical operations. An account of human action that uses the language of data-processing models cannot be adequate unless it recognises possibilities open to the person in human terms. He suggests that the language of cognitive science language treats intentions, beliefs and desires as inaccessible processes, rather than as embodied existential states. For example, Dennett (1978) talks of an 'intentional system' giving a behaviour meaning – but 'intentional' in Dennett's terms includes any system ascribing beliefs, desires and intentions. An experiential level of description is sadly lacking, to the extent that the 'intentional system' is unspecified in the context of static understanding.

Subjective intention and meaning sit unhappily with cognitive science, and are grounded in a very superficial and abstract language of description. The meaning attributed to action and reaction in cognitive-science terms is very different from an ontological analysis of meaning. 'The telic concepts', as Williams notes, 'are taken to be the necessary products of the cognitive system; but they are simply necessary in the sense that brute matter is simply necessary. They obey rational not human laws' (Williams 1987: 212). The phenomena that the clinician observes are complex and experiential and travel across boundaries once considered by experimentalists to be hypothetically distinct. The conspicuously absent component of computer analogue hypotheses is the entity so important to phenomenologists, namely, lived experience.

CONSCIOUSNESS AND UNCONSCIOUSNESS IN COGNITIVE SCIENCE

Summerhoff (1990) offers a technical definition of the faculty of consciousness as the ability of the brain to form an internal representation of the world and self-in-the-world. The latter representation is a complex one in that it monitors the perceptual processing itself. Summerhof outlines three aspects to consciousness: first-order awareness of distal events; a second-order self-awareness; and a third-order reflective awareness of awareness, which accounts for how I am aware that I am aware. We will return to these levels of consciousness, particularly the secondary and tertiary levels, in later chapters.

Many cognitive scientists have placed a great deal of emphasis on the role of verbally-mediated material as the medium through which matured human consciousness is oriented. For example, Guidano (1991) is of the opinion that consciousness is structured through an explicit linguistic ability that 're-orders' and 'scaffolds' self-experience in terms of propositions. As a consequence, explicit restructuring of evaluative judgement makes new levels of abstraction available, transforming the continuous modulation of internal states into patterns for self-understanding, enabling regulation of experience, and facilitation of further reasoning.

Many forms of input data are not, however, immediately verbally coded as propositions which occupy the centre of consciousness; a person may be vaguely aware of strange feelings before they can be verbalised. The literature on subliminal perception shows that subjects can develop preferences for emotional stimuli which are too weak to produce subsequent verbal recognition (Nisbett and De Camp Wilson 1977). Johnson (1988) suggests that much awareness of the world, particularly awareness of sensation, is prelogical and accepted on the basis of faith rather than rationalisation. Cognitive processes come into play only when higher-order critical judgement is required. For instance, subjects may not be able to verbalise the reinforcement contingencies to which they are exposed, while nonetheless responding in a manner suggesting the acquisition of conditioned learning. This 'learning without awareness', as it is called, is quoted by cognitivists and behaviourists alike as an example of the limitations of awareness.

Awareness, it has been said, is unreliable as a guide to understanding motivation and inadequate as an explanation of human behaviour. This latter viewpoint was forcefully put over in a benchmark review paper by Nisbitt and De Camp Wilson (1977) entitled 'Telling more than we can know: Verbal reports on mental processes'. These authors reviewed a wide range of studies, the results of which showed the subjects' lack of ability to report observed influences on their behaviour. Subjects were particularly oblivious to cognitive influences, such as their attributional assumptions. When a response is demonstrated to have been influenced by an experimenter-induced attributional set, subjects denied it, even when presented with the evidence. Furthermore, the subjects gave spurious rationalisations for their actions. There are many examples in which data that influence feeling and behaviour are unconscious, such as subliminal perception, perceptual set and guiding principles or rules, such as syntax. Syntax is an interesting example of unconscious processing, since it is a shared set of rules which profoundly influences verbal behaviour, yet only a minority of people are ever aware of its existence in the sense of gaining the ability to articulate its properties.

Sartre (1943/57) was of the opinion that because conscious experience is limited at any given moment, what we are *not* conscious of is as important as what we are conscious of, in influencing our perception and evaluating. Baars (1988) goes some way to grounding conscious experience within the context of cognitive science, in the process expanding the latter from a limited epistemology; he defines consciousness as the sum total of current awareness. The concept of unconscious events, that is, unexperienced data, is not solely the domain of psychoanalytic theory. We are stating the obvious in order to avoid conceptual confusion over the term 'unconscious'. For Baars, most data in memory, for example, is not currently utilised, and therefore is not experienced in consciousness at a given moment and, hence, is unconscious. He begins by approaching the topic with the premise that conscious awareness at any given moment is remarkably limited when compared with the level of sophistication of human intellectual and biosocial ability. There is ample evidence to support the notion of attention and awareness as self-limiting in the volume of input data which can be processed at any given moment. Miller (1956) provides the classical historic example in his influential article with the self-explanatory title, 'The magical number seven, plus or minus two: Some limits on our capacity for processing information'. Yet the limited capacity to process information at any given moment contrasts sharply with the range of information which is unconsciously stored, and which is potentially accessible. Baars suggests that the limited capacity of attention is functional and has been evolved in order to restrict the amount of information available to consciousness, ensuring that utilised information is contextually appropriate. Contextually-inappropriate information is edited out, and the bottleneck of consciousness, as a limited-capacity channel, ensures that there is a minimum of inappropriate noise in the system.

The implication of this straightforward premise is that consciousness and attention are inextricably bound together, though the relationship between consciousness and attention is a complex one. Baars suggests a model of consciousness which depicts experience and non-experience as a continuum, rather than a simple all-or-none distinction. The gradation of conscious to unconscious events is well established in cognitive science and there are many examples of 'barely attended' percepts. Perhaps the most celebrated of these is the ability to 'shadow' background noise, but orient to it only if personally significant information appears. This happens at a party when one is engrossed in conversation, apparently cutting out the background chatter of other people, until one's own name is mentioned somewhere else in the room. Suddenly, the cited person's ears prick up, demonstrating very clearly that awareness is far from limited to the central focus of attention. This is the aptly-named 'cocktail party phenomenon'.

Consciousness therefore, is more complex than an all-or-none process, so that there are shades of grey between what is conscious and what is not conscious. Baars (1988) has drawn up a list of cognitive events which represent various levels of conscious experience. These range from 'clearly conscious phenomena' to 'clearly unconscious events', with an intermediate level of psychological events which have neither conscious nor unconscious status, the so-called 'fuzzy, difficult-to-determine' events (see Figure 1.1).

Baars classifies consciousness into two basic categories: focal consciousness and peripheral consciousness. Focal consciousness consists of data which is fully attended to, filling the psychological field, such as attended percepts, clear mental images, deliberate inner speech and material deliberately retrieved from memory. The fuzzy difficult-to-determine events include presuppositions and 'subliminal' events which have a subsequent effect on consciousness. Baars makes the point that consciousness is a difficult enough entity without adding complexity at the outset of its study; in any area of scientific enquiry, research should progress from the simplest object of study and progress to the more difficult areas, rather than vice versa. To Baars, this means starting with cognitive processes which are at the centre of a subject's awareness.

> Trying to tackle the most difficult phenomena first is simply destructive of the normal process of science. It leads to confusion and controversy, rather than clarity. When Newton began the modern study of light, he did not begin with the complicated question of wave-particle duality, but with a simple prism and a ray of sunlight.
>
> (Baars 1988)

Therefore, for Baars, clearly conscious phenomena are recommended as the first object of study. Fortunately for Baars, and possibly for psychology in general, this is precisely what cognitive psychologists in the field of mental health have done, using as their starting point the description of the clearly conscious events of their patients, rather than begin with the study of unconscious or barely conscious events.

Clearly conscious phenomena

↑
    Attended percepts
    Clear mental images
    Deliberate inner speech
    Material deliberately retrieved from memory
    Fleeting mental images
    Peripheral or 'background' perceptual events
    Abstract but accessible concepts

Fuzzy, difficult-to-determine events

    Active, but unrehearsed items in immediate memory
    Presuppositions of conscious concepts
    Fully habituated stimuli
    Subliminal events that prime later conscious processes
    'Blind sight' in occipital brain damage
    Contextual information, set
    Automatic skill components
    Unretrieved material in long-term memory
    Perceptual context
↓
    Abstract rules, as syntax

Clearly unconscious events

Figure 1.1   Levels of conscious experience.
Source: B. J. Baars (1988)

THE BIRTH OF COGNITIVE THERAPY

From the 1950s onwards, a group of experienced therapists began suspending their interest in unconscious processes in favour of the more easily observable transparent phenomena. This is particularily true of Albert Ellis and Aaron Beck, both of whom abandoned the psychodynamic model in favour of the (conscious) events of inner speech. Cognitive psychology in the mental health context has its special problems. For cognitive therapists, a legitimate test for whether an event entered consciousness is whether the person can verbally report it (Nisbett and De Camp Wilson 1977; Summerhoff 1990), though it is recognised that elucidation of material is a demanding task. Humanistic psychologists have probably helped in outlining a style of interaction with clients which stresses the necessity of maintaining an ongoing dialogue between clinician and patient. For example, Rogerian counselling demonstrated a method of identifying core assumptions and self-knowledge which are not presented by the patient at first meeting and may serve as a means of rendering assumptions and generalisations on the periphery of consciousness more amenable to vocalisation.

It would be misleading to imagine that cognitive therapy arose out of cognitive science. There are certainly attempts now by therapists to verify clinical hypotheses using cognitive-science paradigms, but this is a current, not historical, liaison. Cognitive therapy developed, on the one hand, from the reaction of Beck and his contemporary Ellis to the dogmas of psychoanalysis, and, on the other hand, from the reaction of Michael Mahoney and his contemporary Donald Meichenbaum and others to the limitations of a strictly behavioural approach, which ignored the mind. All four of these founding fathers accorded more emphasis to the style and content of the client's verbal accounts as legitimate signs of psychopathology in their own right than was allowed in either traditional psychoanalysis or behaviourism.

Mahoney and Lyddon (1988) claim that the intellectual roots from which cognitive therapy arose share the same source as phenomenology; in the eighteenth century, Kant made a distinction between distal stimuli and perception with which modern-day clinical strategies are compatible. Kant discriminated between distal stimuli, which he termed 'noumena' and experience, or 'phenomena'. External objects were described as things-in-themselves, with qualities which are unknowable in terms of their comprehensive physical nature, since matter is not directly transferable into sensation. Experience of a distal object or event occurs by suspending the percept in the context of the subject's prior knowledge and disposition. Evaluation of the percept takes place in this context, the end result of which is an interpretation of the external thing. Things cannot be known as themselves, since only an interpretation of environmental or interoceptive data constitutes experience. It is the construing of events which the cognitive therapist attempts to modify.

There is more than one meaning to the term cognitive activity. The classical use of the term is synonymous with information processing, particularly the processing of data by the human nervous system and computer analogues of the same activities. Cognitive activity is used in a more limited sense by cognitive therapists to refer to conscious activity of a linguistic nature. Rational Emotive Therapy (Ellis 1962) explicitly aims to identify incorrect thought premises and, often, to change maladaptive false assumptions by confrontation. It is in this more limited sense that the conceptualisation of cognitive psychology has entered the field of psychological therapy. Beck (1963, 1976), whose clinical case studies have until recently been largely confined to anxiety and depression, aimed to identify maladaptive assumptions and thought premises and often advocates supplying a competing cognition to derail the maladaptive one. Even so, Kovacs and Beck (1978) viewed cognition as a broad term referring both to the content of thought and the processes involved in thinking; both the processes and the products of knowing.

Mahoney (1991) feels that 'constructivism' is the key element that marks cognitive therapy out from other talking therapies. A crucial cognitive premise is that what the person anticipates, sees and thinks about circumstances and events is distinguishable from the event itself; how an event is evaluated determines the subject's reaction far more than the objective characteristics of the situation. A stimulus event is imbued with meaning in order to make sense of it. In the process, the stimulus event is given an interpretation, so that the percept is elaborated. It is this process of construction of the significance of a stimulus which Mahoney saw to be the core material with which cognitive therapists work. From the outset, cognitive therapists concerned themselves with self-reflection and the evaluation of self in relation to real and anticipated events, of both a somatic and exteroceptive source. The emphasis of cognitive therapy is the content of current consciousness, particularly verbally-mediated material in the form of covert self-statements and, perhaps more importantly, the meaning structures underlying them.

Cognitive therapists have created a culture in which the clinician has started to evolve operational models of psychopathology in information-processing terms. It might seem natural in the future that the cognitive therapist should look to cognitive science for help in constructing clinical cognitive models. Over the past few years, cognitive laboratory studies have began to give empirical confirmation to assumptions which clinical psychologists and psychiatrists practising cognitive therapy had already adopted (see Chapter 2). It will be interesting to see whether laboratory-based studies will aid therapy in the future. There is a growing trend for laboratory-based research to be carried out by cognitive therapists themselves, and this may help steer cognitive science towards the concerns of the clinician.

SUMMARY

The notion of percepts as unique sensory phenomena peculiar to the recipient was born out of the philosophical writings of Kant, to be taken up later by Hegel in his concept of the dialectic reconstruction of distal events. Theoretical interest in idiopathic experience is an integral part of phenomenological thinking. Existential phenomenologists have tended to de-emphasise the Freudian notion of libido as the major volitional component of human experience, in favour of a wider concept, that of the struggle for the unique experience of being. Structural phenomenology, on the other hand, has attempted the analysis of human experience within a more specific framework of awareness, studying consciousness both in terms of its content and, more importantly, its form.

Cognitive therapy can be viewed as a structural phenomenological approach to the content of conscious experience, in that cognitive therapists are interested in subjective experience and try to make sense of it by an inductive and deductive approach to the exposed self-world data. For example, in clinical anxiety, cognitive therapists find that patients consistently assess the world as posing more threat than is borne out by fact, and assess the self as being helplessly unable to cope with the consequences of such worldly threats. Cognitive therapists largely concentrate on modifying interpretations of self and world by challenging beliefs and externalising barely articulated but incorrect assumptions and propositions.

Chapter 2

The relationship between feeling and thought

Traditionally, thought and feeling have been considered separate but related areas. The exact nature of the relation has recently sparked major controversies between Lazarus and Zajonc. Lazarus (1984), in line with a view popular within the cognitive therapy movement, maintains that thoughts can control feeling and that appraisal triggers emotions. Zajonc (1984) argues that thoughts are always immersed in feelings, and that emotions precede and activate cognitions. Watts (1990) has argued that feelings are independent of thought but induce special feeling-related cognitions. These alternative views raise a crucial question, namely, are the 'feeling self' and the 'thinking self' two separate experiences?

Clarification of the relatedness of thought and feeling is crucial in defining the core concept of 'self' in cognitive psychology. Izard (1979) views self as the product of the interaction of emotional and cognitive systems. He postulates that these systems, 'necessarily share neural circuits of interconnecting neural pathways to allow the systems to develop as the holistic set that we identify as the individual, autonomous person' (Izard 1979: 17). The implication is that, though emotion and cognition can be separated at a conceptual level, in everyday functioning, 'the emotional system and the cognitive system interact in intricate and complex ways in facilitating the integration of the super system, or individual person, and in bonding of person to person in social relationships' (ibid.: 18). It follows from this model that a dysfunction in either the emotional or cognitive systems may result in problems pertaining to self-concept and self-awareness. Izard illustrates ways in which the interdependence of emotion and cognition occurs.

For Izard (1979, 1991), emotion enters the psychological field, at a conscious level, as feeling, with no cognitive component. Subsequently, the feeling is accompanied by cognitive evaluation, forming a cognitive-affective structure. The cognitive overlay is the product of socio-cultural learning and experience. It is these cognitive-affective structures which, for Izard, form the basis of self. As we shall see later, particularly in Chapter 6, disruption of the feeling quality of an experience can have ramifications for self-awareness, to the extent that if the feeling self is not operational in an emotionally-charged situation, feelings of unreality may result. Conversely, if the cognitive evaluation of a feeling or sensation is distorted, the subsequent emotional state may have a detrimental effect on self-concept, a state of affairs which can be extremely disruptive for the individual concerned (for example, see Chapter 4 on self-concept in relation to panic disorder).

This chapter is concerned with a limited aspect of the cognitive-emotional system, namely, the relationship between thought and feeling. For present purposes we will differentiate between feeling and emotion in much the same way as Izard: while emotion is a combination of affective and intellectual processes, feeling reflects an irreducible affective state, which is usually enriched by rationale and personal meaning in retrospect to the feeling state itself.

On the face of it, thought and feeling seem to go hand in hand, and are inextricably bound together. Yet unless the interface between thought and feeling is explored, and their relatedness explored, this 'nearness' remains based more on intuition and philosophical debate than on scientific fact. There are serious linguistic, philosophical and empirical problems which shroud the theories and research pertaining to the interface between feeling and other processes affecting the psychological field. One such problem is whether or not feeling can be isolated in some sort of pure unattached form, irrespective and independent of the verbal encoding, concept formation and self-awareness which accompanies it.

WHAT IS FEELING?

Conceptually, feeling is understood only loosely, perhaps more by intuition than by formal, watertight definition. Jaspers makes the following comment:

> Commonly the term 'feeling' is given to any psychic event that clearly does not belong to the phenomena of object awareness, nor to instinctual excitation and volitional acts. All undeveloped, undefined psychic manifestations tend to get called 'feeling'. That is, everything intangible, analytically elusive, everything for which we can find no other name. Someone feels he does not care, or that something is not right. He feels that the room is too small or that everything is clear or he feels uneasy, etc. This diverse set of phenomena which we term 'feelings' has never been satisfactorily analysed from the psychological point of view. We do not know what constitutes the basic elements nor do we know how to classify (feeling).
>
> (Jaspers 1963: 108)

For Jaspers, feelings reflect the sensation of internal atmosphere. Referring to the range of pathological feelings, Jaspers suggests a typology of abnormal feeling states which can be divided up as follows: apathy, feelings of personal incapacity, changes in the feeling tone of perception (including changes in bodily feelings), and the feeling of having lost feeling. Of particular interest to us here are the changes in feelings of capacity, which correspond approximately to the notion of 'self-efficacy'. Whilst Lazarus (1984) views self-efficacy as a product of verbally-mediated judgement, Jaspers (1963) suggests otherwise. For Jaspers, an introspective impression of personal resourcefulness arises from an intuitive, non-verbal source.

About feelings of capacity, Jaspers has the following to say:

We always have some feeling of our capacity; this gives us confidence in ourselves without any explicit awareness of the underlying feeling. In depression, patients get a feeling of insufficiency, one of their most common complaints. In part these feelings are of real insufficiency and in part they are unfounded, primary feelings. Awareness of being useless for the real world, of being incompetent and incapable of action, of being unable to make a decision, of wavering, of being clumsy, of not being able to think or understand anymore, all these are the burden of many abnormal states, though real inefficiency need not exist.

(Jaspers 1963: 111)

In the above quotation, Jaspers appears to draw a distinction between feelings related to objective external fact ('an awareness of real insufficiency'), and feelings unrelated to the external world ('unfounded primary feelings'). Jaspers's use of the word 'primary' carries the implication that a feeling of insufficiency can emerge independently of verbally-mediated processes, manifesting itself in some sort of pure unadulterated form as a negative, but unarticulated, sensory impression of self-awareness.

The idea of unattached feelings is viewed with considerable scepticism by many psychotherapists of diverse persuasions. Some cognitive therapists insist that feeling is inevitably set within an evaluative context and a pre-existing framework of expectations, which systematically guide attention towards a limited experiential range of affect. The latter is inextricably linked to self-image and propositional self-statements in the form of self-dialogue. Where these are not obvious, cognitive therapists have proposed that the cognitive processes are 'barely conscious' or outside of the current range of consciousness. In contrast to Jaspers, Lazarus' view is that without prior appraisal, feeling cannot exist.

The notion of fleeting, barely conscious thoughts and images is supported by the early psychologist and philosopher William James (1890) and, more recently, by cognitive scientists such as Baars (1988). For cognitive therapists, feelings of insufficiency are not 'primary', but arise out of a complex process of evaluation, whether such higher-order processes are immediately evident or not. Self-image, or self-concept, is considered to underlie all feelings of insufficiency. Insufficiency feelings are therefore viewed as arising within a wider psychological epistemological context.

An implication of Jaspers's irreducibility premise is that the feeling, which is devoid of thinking, provokes cognitions which arise in retrospect, when the subject searches for a meaning to the feeling:

The elementary breakthrough of experiences, which are not understandable in their genesis, is manifested in unattached feelings. If they become meaningful to the subject, these feelings must first search for an object or try to create one. The feelings simply arise in the first place and remain in force though they may never find an object. For instance, unattached anxiety is very common in depressive states, so is contentless euphoria in manic states, so is obscure erotic excitement in puberty, so are the feelings roused in the early stages of pregnancy and in the early stages of a psychosis. Driven by an almost inescapable need to give some content to such feelings, patients will often supply some such content on their own. It is a sign of critical insight if feelings are actually described as lacking in content.

(Jaspers 1963: 13)

However, as we shall see later, laboratory evidence would suggest that the content of thought during a given feeling state is not deliberately and voluntarily constructed to fit a prevailing feeling state, but is automatic, in that feeling excites specific memory nodes and linguistic processing channels involuntarily.

The terms 'mood', 'affect', 'feeling' and 'emotion' are interrelated and broadly encompass a series of qualitative states of being. It is often said that the hedonic tone of such states is partly a reflection of the degree of differentiation and interpretation accorded by the subject. According to this view, experientially, feeling is said to emanate from an undifferentiated internal state, which then becomes subject to cognitive enrichment.

The cognitive therapy movement has proved reluctant to accept the premise that the differentiation of feeling arises independently of thought, and has challenged the notion of the irreducibility of feeling. This is because many affective shifts are attributable to thoughts, attitudes and cognitive schemata. Some cognitive theorists go as far as to say that there is only one feeling state, that of arousal; the ensuing experience is then said to be shaped by its cognitive enrichment, which arises from such factors as self-concept and attributional interpretation pertaining to what the arousal really means (Bentall 1993, personal communication).

However, thought and feeling are not inseparable. Watts (1992) provides an example in which the role of thinking is minimal in constituting an aberrant emotional experience, in that retarded depression typically involves a paucity of thought. Some authors prefer to make a temporal distinction between thought and feeling, with important implications for causality.

The issue of causality remains unresolved and the relative influence of thought over feeling is controversial. Zajonc's (1984) position, that feeling states are primary and become transformed into thoughts, of feeling-congruent content, is related to Jaspers's notion of unanchored affect, which only in retrospect to its experience is supplied with a propositional rationale. There is some evidence in support of Zajonc's affective primacy hypothesis from commonplace observations in everyday life – an angry person who brings the anger affect into a neutral situation often harbours critical thoughts and sentiments of irritation towards an innocent party. Though the new object of criticism and irritation may be totally inoffensive in objective terms, the angry person is influenced by his/her prevailing mood and finds that thoughts of resentment and dislike readily appear, backed by self-justification, despite the absence of provocation by the innocent recipient.

The view that thinking can precipitate feelings (e.g. Lazarus 1984b) is a direction of causality, which is provided support by Velten (1968) in what has become a celebrated experimental procedure. Velten induced specific self-referential propositions, by getting subjects to read out loud a series of either negative or positive self-statements. Subsequent mood changed in direction accordingly, depending on whether the subject had read out self-derogating or positive self-statements. In reality, the question of whether feeling or thought is primary is an impossible one, not least because from the moment of waking, in the natural flow of events, there is a constant interplay between linguistic processing and affective state. Nonetheless, attempts have been made to modify emotion experimentally, by temporarily depriving the subject of thinking activity, by discontinuing linguistic processing while an emotion is taking place. Some of the major research findings using this methodological approach are provided below.

THE EFFECTS OF UNATTACHED FEELING ON THINKING

Methodological problems in research investigating the relationship between thinking and feeling are inevitable, since the appraisal of feeling is usually based upon criteria which are self-evaluative, such as assessment of self-worth, projected competence and coping abilities. These self-referential criteria of 'feelings', used particularly in the measurement of depression or anxiety, are therefore not pure in Jaspers' sense of unattached feelings, but, rather, the name of the feeling is inferred from self-judgemental criteria. It is difficult to escape from self-evaluative statements as a criterion of depressed mood. Therefore, much of the research into the interrelationship of thought and feeling is tautological, in that the ostensibly separate dependent and independent variables overlap considerably. When mood is investigated as the causative factor in shaping content of thought, the mood state itself is normally measured in terms of verbally-mediated material. For example, the feeling of sadness is characteristically defined in terms of pessimistic outlook.

However, in a series of ingenious experiments carried out by Bower *et al.* (1978), linguistically-unattached feeling states of happiness, sadness, fear and anger were elicited with the use of an hypnotic procedure. The notable aspect of this experimental procedure is that while the feeling state is brought about by eliciting mood-inducing thoughts by use of the Velten procedure, Bower *et al.* then discontinued the conscious mood-inducing thoughts so that the mood state occurred in the absence of accompanying propositional statements. These experiments serve to investigate the development of conscious thought and information processing from a position of primary affect, i.e. from a feeling state devoid of an accompanying reference point. Their general procedure was as follows.

An hypnotic-suggestibility scale was administered to a non-clinical population, consisting of university students and staff. The highest 15 per cent of scorers were then selected to undergo the hypnotic induction procedure described by Weitzenhoffer and Hilgard (1962). Subjects were then instructed to recall vividly a series of personal experiences of either an exclusively happy or sad nature. Once the required mood had been established, each subject was instructed to forget the specific emotionally-laden memory which had triggered the corresponding mood. Still under hypnosis, the subjects were then instructed to retain the same mood state, which was subsequently accentuated by getting the subjects to focus on the feeling which had been elicited. Thus, a 'free-floating' affective state, detached from the Velten-style procedure by which it was induced, was accentuated. This procedure formed the basis from which a series of information-processing experiments were constructed.

In one of the first of the series, Bower and Gilligan (1980) requested their subjects to complete a diary of happy and sad events which occurred during a normal working week and evaluate their intensity. On their return to the experimental situation, Bower and Gilligan induced happy and sad mood states in each subject, in accordance with the procedure described above. During each of the induced moods, each subject was then asked to re-recall the events of the previous week and to rate the intensity of feeling associated with them. Subjects in a pleasant mood recalled more happy recent experiences than unhappy ones (31 per cent pleasant, 23 per cent unpleasant), while in the induced sad mood the reverse was observed (38 per cent unpleasant, and 33 per cent pleasant). It is interesting to note that the percentage of pleasant recent experiences recalled remained the same under both mood conditions, but the percentage of unpleasant experiences recalled increased appreciably. Assuming that the results of experimentally-induced mood can be generalised for patients with affective disorder, the results would suggest that depressed individuals can be characterised by their relative ease of recall of negative events (with approximately 15 per cent greater ease than pleasant events in the Bower and Gilligan study).

During the same procedure, subjects were asked to re-evaluate previously-recalled biographical events in terms of the degree of happiness/sadness associated with them. During the induced pleasant mood condition, subjects tended to rate happy events as even happier and sad events as less sad than in the initial rating, thus making light of painful memories. By contrast, during the induced sad mood there was a change in retrospective evaluation in the opposite direction, with subjects recalling happy events as less happy, while exaggerating the intensity of unhappy memories by rating them as far more unhappy than in the pre-experiment rating. The effect of amplification of mood state is therefore seen not only to render aberrant mood-congruent memories more available, but also results in a re-evaluation of those memories, distorting recall with an accentuated positive or negative evaluative tone. This work suggests that change in mood is a determinant of the judgement of retrospective events.

In a further experiment, Monteiro and Bower (1980) investigated the effect of mood on remote memory, during conditions of experimentally-induced happiness and sadness. Subjects were asked to free-recall childhood events. In the 'happy' condition, almost all of the vignettes provided by the subjects were judged as pleasant, while subjects rendered sad by the hypnotic procedure provided more vignettes from remote memory which were sad. (Ratings of the hedonic flavour of the vignettes were derived from the subjects themselves later, while in a neutral mood.)

The data illustrate that mood has the effect of producing selective recall and also influences the retrospective judgement of events, shedding some light on the internal world of subjects with altered affect: current mood selectively mars recall of opposite-flavoured events, while rendering mood-congruent events more accessible. In effect, the depressed subject is partially blinded to light-hearted aspects of his/her history by virtue of the pattern of retrieval brought into play by the predominant affect. Such findings raise the question of whether knowledge of such mechanisms can inspire a clinical means of short-circuiting this apparently circular process. Two important issues concerning depressed patients are: first, how distorted retrospective evaluation can be altered; and, second, whether memories of a non-depressive content can be accessed in order to escape total submergence within a meaning-matrix of overwhelming negativity.

State-dependent learning as a mechanism of mood-congruent distortion of memory

It is well established that recall is enhanced when the environmental cues present during the acquisition stage of learning are also present during the period in which the recall takes place. For example, Abernathy (1940) found that students taking their final examinations in the room in which they had been taught achieved a higher standard than students who were examined in a different room. This effect is thought to be due to environmental factors acting as cues, prompting recall and making stored information more accessible. In an experiment involving the same subjects under varied conditions, Godden and Baddeley (1975) got deep-sea divers to learn lists of words on the deck of their boat and underwater. Their findings indicated that recall was superior when it took place in a situation similar to that in which the original acquisition of the information took place, whether it be underwater or on the surface of the ocean.

The enhancement of recall by the presence of the same cues as in the learning situation is not just limited to environmental factors. In an experiment investigating the effects of marijuana, Eich (1980) found that memory for words was more accessible if recall was requested during the same state as that in which learning had occurred, whether it be 'marijuana-intoxicated' or 'no intoxication'. In other words, a greater amount of material learned during cannabis intoxication is recalled during marijuana intoxication than when 'straight' and vice versa.

The same state-dependent effect has been noted with alcohol (Parker *et al.* 1976). This perhaps points to some of the difficulties of combating the craving for alcohol, apart from the withdrawal reactions, in long-term alcohol abuse; cessation of the habit may reduce recall of the everyday life events which took place during the (often prolonged) period of abuse and hence detract from the continuity of identity. It is feasible that withdrawing subjects are prompted back into substance abuse partly because the events learned during a prolonged period of intoxication become inaccessible during sobriety. Unfortunately, returning to alcohol then becomes the easiest and most direct route back to a meaningful existence, since recall of recent events (presumably including emotional recall) is thereby enhanced.

The notion of state-dependent recall has some interesting implications for everyday life experience, should the above results be generalisable, in terms of more naturally elicited affect and more true-to-life content of learning. It would be predicted, for example, that material learned while depressed would be recalled with difficulty in a subsequent non-depressed mood. Following a recovery from a depressive episode, this would presumably have advantages, in compartmentalising sad memories, breaking an otherwise circular pattern of depressed mood–depressed thought–depressed mood; a mood shift towards positive affect would render the pattern of cognitive rehearsal which took place during the depressed period as relatively inaccessible, making it easier to 'jolly oneself along' with nostalgic reminiscences.

This prediction is supported by Henry et al. (1973), using naturally occurring mood swings in bi-polar affective disorder (manic depression). Different word-association lists were presented to manic-depressive patients during the hypomanic and depressive phases. When required to recall word associations, the associations recalled best were those learned in the same mood, though recognition performance was not state-dependent.

Bower (1981) examined the selectivity of mood-dependent learning when the recall mood was dissimilar but not opposite to the mood in which learning took place. Subjects were required to learn a word list in an hypnotically-induced state of either happiness or sadness, or anger or fear. These mood states were chosen to be consistent with Plutchick's (1980) conceptualisation of emotion. Plutchick views both happiness and sadness and anger and fear as diametrically opposite pairs. When the subjects were asked to recall the list in the same mood as the learning condition, Bower found recall scores averaged 85 per cent. When the recall mood was opposite to that of the learning condition, recall averaged 54 per cent, indicating that mood is a potent cue of recall; at least as potent as cues from an external source. Bower then went on to measure recall in a mood which was dissimilar, but not opposite to the learning condition (for example, learn during happiness or sadness, recall during anger or fear); recall during a dissimilar but not opposite mood averaged 70 per cent, a lower performance than when learning and recall occurred in the same mood state, but appreciably higher than recall in a mood opposite to that in which learning occurred.

Clinical implications of mood-determined content of consciousness

The above research implicates mood as a profound influence on thinking. If the sample of experimental findings above are generalisable to emotional disorders, the following points are of particular clinical relevance:

(a) while suffering from an affective disorder, the most accessible memories are those which are compatible in content with the affect concerned

(b) Such recall is likely to distort self-referential material and maintain the dysfunction

(c) The most inaccessible memories are those which are incongruent with the emotional dysfunction. These are the memories which would be the most likely to regulate the emotion concerned, if they could be accessed readily

(d) Interruption of an emotional dysfunction is rendered difficult by virtue of the ease of availability of distorted, mood-corrupted cognition and the inaccessibility of thought representative of the opposite mood. Information relating to the latter is poorly recalled during the dysfunctional state

(e) Subjects are more receptive to cognitions pertaining to an adaptive mood which is unrelated but not opposite to the emotional dysfunction than cognitions representative of opposing mood

THE INFLUENCE OF THINKING ON FEELING

In the summary above, we have made two important assumptions: first, that depressed patients, by virtue of their cognitive operations, exhibit a consciousness which is flooded with negative thoughts and images; and, second, that negative thoughts and images are detrimental to mood, acting as feed-forward cues of further affective disturbance. This latter claim, concerning the feed-forward properties of cognitions, is now considered.

The evidence that thought and vocalisation influence emotion is substantial. Velten (1968) got a series of non-clinical subjects to read out statements, the content of which involved themes of either personal success and good fortune, or of glumness, personal failure and inadequacy. Content had a significant effect on mood, in that subsequent to the reading of the positive self-statements, subjects exhibited a mood shift towards elation, while the reading of the series of negative self-statements had the opposite effect. Such findings underpin a major assumption of cognitive therapy, that is, that the content of cognitions, in the form of self-talk, selectively induces affective states, whether they be adaptive or dysfunctional. A rationale underlying cognitive therapy is that any mood is preceded by the cognitive events which have brought the affect into play. If the affect is detrimental to the beholder, it can be manipulated by changing thinking with a view to eliciting an emotional configuration that will be more adaptive and will block the aberrant affective state. Cognition is thus seen to be the independent variable, while emotion is seen to be the consequence, or the dependent variable.

In a sample of fifty depressed patients, Beck (1963) found a number of trends in the content of thought which differentiated the clinical group from non-clinical controls. The typical statements of the patient group were coloured with a sense of hopelessness about the future, predictions of personal failure and excessive self-criticism. Self-evaluation was characterised by an unrealistically low assessment of abilities and an equally low self-worth. Though Beck initially trained as a psychoanalyst, he began to feel with increasing conviction that the pattern of statements uttered by his patients did not fit the pattern predicted by pyschoanalytic theory and that self-concept was of major importance in maintaining the affective disorder. In any case, Beck viewed psychodynamic psychotherapy as an obscure route to the underlying meaning structures. Beck began to develop the conviction that the utterances of his patients were highly systematised and the forms predictable in ways which psychodynamic theory left unexplained. As a result, Beck moved away from his initial psychoanalytic orientation.

Beck appreciated that self-concept was an important feature of self-talk and that anxiety and depression could be identified by the respective self-evaluative cognitions which accompanied them. Rather than view negative self-evaluation as a *product* of anxiety and depression, Beck saw evaluative judgements as intrinsic to *maintaining* these problematic states. The flavour of self-assessment appeared to Beck to form a consistent pattern both within and between patients, and therefore Beck proposed that underlying a series of discrete anxious or depressed cognitions was a stable, barely conscious and systematic evaluative template of assumptions, against which events are appraised. He termed these underlying (i.e. barely verbalised, relatively more abstract) general assumptions meta-cognitions or 'schemas'. The major tasks of cognitive therapy became two-fold: first, modification of cognitions congruent with the negative, ahedonic state; second, the delineation, that is, the exposure into full consciousness, of the self-concept, for the purpose of changing abstract notions about worth, capability and so on.

That is not to say Beck defined depression in terms of thought processes alone, since he also considered depressive phenomena in terms of neurophysiological processes at the neurotransmitter level. His hypotheses about the aetiology of depression are multi-modal and this is reflected in his clinical intervention strategies, which include both the modification of self-appraisal and expectation (cognitive) and medication, particularly the tricyclic antidepressants (pharmacological). Recent studies have led Beck to emphasise the cognitive aspects of therapy far more than pharmacological intervention, since a comparison of both treatment approaches in depression resulted in a relatively more favourable response to the former (Beck *et al.* 1985).

The hallmark of Beck's earlier work was the identification of the '*Einstellung*', or 'fixedness' of the negative thinking of depressed patients. It should be added that the information-processing mechanisms underlying the circularity of depressed patients were developed and acquired empirical support subsequent to clinical observation. Beck has become a figurehead of cognitive therapy, though other distinguished clinicians also outlined self-appraisal and self-efficacy as the major problem area to be targeted in therapy, including Lazarus (1991) and Bandura (1977).

The organisation of cognition: schemata

One of Beck's most acknowledged contributions to the cognitive literature was his attempt to account for the organisation of an individual's psychological make-up in terms of a structural mechanism. This mechanism, underlying surface cognitions, moods and patterns of behaviour was depicted in terms of 'schemas', or 'schemata', concepts which exemplify the attempt by the therapy fraternity to create a theoretical framework of direct clinical relevance. In this instance, Beck's aim was not description, but explanation of the enduring nature of psychological dysfunction.

The concept of schema (or schemata) was first used by Piaget, in the 1920s, to explain the rules of perceptual organisation and interpretation during child development, and was later borrowed by Beck (1976). Beck felt that the consistency of bias judgement associated with clinical problems implied the existence of a cognitive structure around which judgements were organised. Schemata refer to the way in which subjective evaluative activity is structured to give meaning to events and to integrate information. Their content may refer to self (including interoceptive stimuli and self-concept), to others, or may have an impersonal content, such as with the evaluation of external objects, events or abstract concepts. Beck outlined a number of the properties of schemata. First, they vary in breadth of scope, so that some are more all-embracing than others. Second, schemata can be either psychoactive or latent in their influence on the judgement and prioritisation of attention at any one time. When a schema is 'hypervalent' it takes on a prominent position in the psychological field, displacing the influence of other schemata.

Beck *et al.* (1990) felt that schemata are comparable with Kelly's personal constructs (Kelly 1955). The similarity lies in the function that these conceptual structures have: both serve to make sense of the world by prioritising personally-significant criteria; both influence the information processing of circumstances in which the subject finds him/herself. Schematisation and construing have a direct effect on information processing from start to finish. By determining the priority which competing distal stimuli are given, the focus of attention is directed substantially by hypervalent schemata. The content of awareness at any given moment is construed within the frame of reference in which the schemata is embedded, affecting both judgement and action.

Beck *et al.* (1990) has made an attempt at classifying schemata, according to the content and functional mode of operation. Affective schemata are implicated in generating feelings, while cognitive schemata are involved in interpretation, abstraction and recall; action plans are organised around instrumental schemas; control schemas direct and monitor actions. Other authors have concentrated on more specific issues of cognitive organisation, using alternative, but compatible concepts.

Lazarus (1991) identified two areas of erroneous judgement which he felt to be of pathogenic significance, namely, primary and secondary appraisal. Primary appraisal involves an evaluation process of central interest to the majority of cognitive theorists, that is, the individual's assessment of the degree of threat in a given situation. Lazarus emphasises that the differences between people requiring clinical help and those who do not lie in the over-inclusiveness of the threatening category when evaluating external events, so that patients requiring therapy were seen by Lazarus as having an unrealistically low threshold to danger. Secondary appraisal refers to the assessment of factors relating to the individual's ability to be instrumental in controlling the threatening circumstances. Secondary appraisal is therefore a reflection of the subject's anticipated ability to cope. Clinically-anxious patients are characterised by biased negative judgement concerning their own personal resources, both in terms of anticipating failure to deal with external events successfully and by envisaging ego collapse or uncontrollable physiological response to the perceived threat.

The clinical implication is that there are two areas of potential change: first, the patient's discriminative judgement regarding which situations pose a threat and which are 'safe'; second, given a situation identified as threatening, the judgement of whether the subject possesses the means to cope sufficiently to regain a position of 'safety'. Modification of secondary appraisal involves the strengthening of both perceived and real coping skills. Lazarus was concerned to modify anticipatory cognitions in such a way that intervention introduced less morbid and pessimistic expectations when dealing with perceived threat. Secondary appraisals inevitably engage self-schemata, particularly those which Beck et al. term 'instrumental schemas' (1990: 33), which involve aspects of the self-concept representing the perceived resourcefulness of coping behaviours.

Watts (1992) suggests that the modification of schemata requires the application of a different set of principles to the modification of surface propositional phenomena, though he does not specify these differences. Propositional phenomena are generally defined as discreet predictive statements regarding the likelihood of a specific outcome. One such approach is the manipulation of expectation. It is common for depressed patients to anticipate the occurrence of negative events in the future. Moreover, subjects experiencing even a transitory depressed mood have a tendency to project into the future in a self-defeating manner, so that there is a general estimation of gloom and negative outcome (Wright and Bower 1981). If expectancy is so self-defeating, it is not difficult to see why severely-depressed patients find engaging in everyday events so difficult, since their subjective appraisal is steeped in failure and despair, corresponding to conditions which Seligman (1975) describes as a component of 'learned helplessness'.

For Beck et al. (1988, 1990), an activated schema generates spontaneous thoughts and imagery of a content which is congruent with the schema itself. These spontaneous cognitions are referred to as 'automatic thoughts'. The automaticity of thinking during anxiety and depression is considered a crucial aspect of these disorders. Automaticity implies that a pattern of tram-line thinking is in operation, whereby the subject has difficulty in scanning the full range of potential evaluative options in the repertoire of thought; the content of consciousness becomes mood-specific and there is considerable difficulty in accessing a wider perspective. The restriction of judgement is not, however, appreciated by the beholder, to whom perception of the world and of him/herself seems logical and conclusive. The restrictiveness of the prevailing cognitive activity prevents the subject from moderating this tunnel vision by adopting a different standpoint; the subject becomes locked within a limited and distorted perspective.

Not all individuals are prone to affective deterioration, even when exposed to an apparently similar level of failure and loss. It is therefore pertinent to enquire about the factors which will render one individual depressed, while another exhibits apparent immunity. If the conditions promoting immunity were known, there would be potential for the depression-prone to acquire the internal characteristics or environmental conditions of the depression-immune. Of relevance to this issue is the question of whether negative automatic thoughts occur in the non-clinical population, or whether they are unique to depressive individuals.

In a recent study, Kumari and Blackburn (1992) obtained cognitive data of twenty-seven non-clinical subjects trained to record negative automatic thoughts over a two-week period, using the Automatic Thoughts Questionnaire (Hollan and Kendall 1980) and the Daily Record of Dysfunctional Thoughts (Beck *et al.* 1979), together with self-ratings of mood state (BDI and STAI). They were then able to compare their results with those derived from depressed patients, the data having been derived by a similar procedure carried out by Blackburn and Evunson (1989). Kumari and Blackburn found that non-clinical control subjects are also prone to distorted thinking, but that there were characteristics distinguishing them from depressed subjects. Whereas the patient sample exhibited thoughts of low self-worth and failure in response to affective swings involving anxiety and depression, the normal subject had a tendency to record thoughts of being frustrated and hard done by, with relatively well-preserved self-worth and externally-directed hostility. As Kumari and Blackburn (1992) point out, their results are consistent with the hypothesis that depressed people exhibit inner-directed hostility, while the non-depressed externalise their anger.

THE PROBLEM OF EMOTIONAL POVERTY

Nemiah *et al.* report that in some clients anxiety states are characterized by 'alexithymia', that is, an inability to describe feelings: 'patients are often unable to localize affects in their bodies and appear unaware of any of the common automatic somatic reactions that accompany the experience of a variety of feelings' (Nemiah *et al.* 1976). Alexithymia is both an affect-deficit disorder and a continuous personality variable (Horton *et al.* 1992). Sifneos (1972) originally identified an inability to describe feelings and an absence of emotional inner life as a platform from which psychosomatic symptoms are likely to emerge. Sifneos suggests that when a general sense of dysphoria occurs in the absence of reciprocal feeling states, the dysphoria focuses on bodily sensations of a physical nature, which form a rationale for the predominantly ahedonic tone. Horton *et al.* (1992), however, have recently applied the Toronto Alexithymia Scale to a normal adolescent population and reported justification for conceptualising the disorder in terms of a personality trait, because of its stability over time. Interestingly, there seems to be an asymmetry between the negative and positive expressions of emotion, since alexithymics are less able to express positive affect than negative affect. Lesser (1985) was impressed by the lack of feeling quality in some patients, particularly those who present with psychosomatic complaints. These patients are often unable to describe the quality of their distress, but nonetheless are dissatisfied by what amounts to a vague absence of well-being.

Alexithymics typically exhibit a stultified fantasy life and are unable to express themselves emotionally. Verbal expression of emotion is impoverished and, importantly, the patient cannot discriminate between various feeling states. This may mean that feelings occur but fail to be enriched with additional (verbal) content, or that the only feeling state which is appreciated as a 'lived-in' experience is a totally undifferentiated ahedonic state. Certainly, alexithymics cannot discriminate between feelings and physical sensations. They complain of somatic sensations in situations which might normally be expected to provoke an emotional response. This unusual and interesting state may prove useful phenomenologically in the consideration of the role of affective and cognitive schemata. However, currently there is no consensus view among cognitive psychologists regarding the source of the affective deficit, particularly on whether the deficit is of an affective or verbal-cognitive nature (i.e. absence of feeling versus failure to identify feeling).

The obscure relationship between cognition and emotion is particularly underlined in depression. This is especially so in severe rather than mild–moderate depression. Severely depressed patients express an indifference and passive resignation to external events. Watts comments:

> Rather than interpreting life-events as having negative meaning, some depressed patients apparently fail to find any personal meaning at all in life events. At a cognitive level, their thoughts show an emphasis, not so much on the negative features of self, world and future, as on their emptiness and meaninglessness.
>
> (Watts 1992)

This may explain why patients, when severely depressed, are not generally a suicide risk and why the risk increases during the initial phases of recovery. One of the major hypotheses for the increased risk is that during partial recovery, events reacquire meaning (albeit negative meaning). Volition prompts the patient to act, whereas in a more severe depressive state, meaninglessness produces a vacuum of goal-directed activity.

The paucity of thinking in retarded depression poses problems for models which propose that feeling states are maintained by cognitive activity. While the principle of parsimony of mood and a hedonic tone of thinking appears to be confirmed for mild to moderate depression, severe depression, with the characteristic loss of concentration and diminution of awareness, does not correspond to any current cognitive model of affective disorder. This will no doubt provide a considerable challenge for cognitive theorists and therapists. A major stumbling block for cognitive therapists faced with the severely depressed patient is the development of rapport, since such patients are often at best monosyllabic and lack spontaneity. Under these conditions, it becomes extremely difficult for the therapist to facilitate the patient's access to mood-incongruent (i.e. non-depressive) information stored in memory. Nihilistic delusions are also a major block to cognitive structuring; when the patient holds the conviction that everything is finished, that the world no longer exists or that the patient him/herself is an empty shell which has degenerated into almost total decay, there is little scope for cognitive restructuring. However, therapists are beginning to construct treatment packages at this more severe extreme of affective dysfunction. Attempts at treatment must incorporate behavioural change and stimulation as a prerequisite of cognitive reshaping (Lazarus 1991).

SUMMARY

Feeling and emotion are lay terms, which are ambiguous and open to interpretation. Some psychological theorists use the terms to distinguish between two distinct levels of affective process. All emotions involve feeling, but while a feeling state comprises an internal atmosphere of affective tone, which inspires imagery and verbally-mediated thinking in retrospect, an emotion contains referents, giving the experience contextual meaning and cognitive enrichment. An emotion is therefore a relatively more structured experiential phenomenon, which will be discussed further in the subsequent chapters. In this chapter, we have concentrated on the relationship between two components of emotion, namely, feeling and thought.

The relationship between thinking and feeling is a bi-directional one. Attending to specific propositions, particularly with reference to the self, have a profound effect on mood. Low self-image, as reflected by description of self-worth and self-efficacy, for example, reduces the hedonic tone of experience, not least because self-image becomes integrated into the evaluation of one's acceptance to others and degree of usefulness. Conversely, experimentally-induced free-floating mood is known to affect self-propositional statements and it would appear that mood 'cues in' particular areas of recall which match the mood, so that for example, a prevailing mood of sadness renders the recall of sad material easier than that of happy memories. Mood-congruent memories are far more accessible than mood-incongruent memories. Such observations are important cornerstones of the cognitive approach to anxiety and depression, since they demonstrate the circularity by which anxious and depressive experience is maintained. However, at the extreme end of the depressive spectrum, the basic tenet that negative self-statements maintain lowered mood does not hold, since severe depression is characterised by a marked absence of self-statements.

There is a trend towards some cognitive therapists developing their own models of information processing, concepts from which are intended for use in the clinical setting. One such concept is the notion of schemata, which are said to represent the organisation of judgements, affect, instrumental plans and strategic action. There is an implication from Beck *et al.*'s (1990) recent publications that schemata from different modalities influence each other, in such a way that they are synchronous, a theoretical observation which is given support by empirical work demonstrating the congruence of mood and themes of thought.

Chapter 3

The problem of defining the moods and emotions

MODELS OF EMOTIONAL EXISTENCE

Sometimes the lay public refer to psychological problems as 'emotional' problems, implying that the emotionality of an individual is at the core of the psychological dysfunction. However, though no clinician would deny the presence of an emotional component to psychogenic reactions, there is little consensus in the literature concerning the nature and breadth of emotion as a concept.

THE EXISTENTIAL PERSPECTIVE ON EMOTION

The emotions have been approached somewhat obliquely by existential phenomenologists. Heidegger (1927) uses the term '*Benfindlichkeit*' to refer to the emotional tone at any given moment. The term translates into English as 'the way one finds oneself'. Macquarrie distinguishes between positive and negative emotions. By negative emotions, he refers to emotions 'which disclose situations we are "already in", so to speak, but where we do not really belong and we want to extricate ourselves or change the pattern of the situation' (Macquarrie 1972). Positive emotions, on the other hand, 'evince a sense of belonging and place a favourable interpretation on the situations that evoke them' (ibid.). This gives emotion a functional aspect in the development of a qualitative reaction to data in awareness. The volitional function of emotion is of central concern to the evolutionary, hard-wired theories which will be mentioned later.

In the existential literature, the negative emotions have recieved more attention than the positive emotions. The twentieth-century existentialists such as Sartre and Heidegger, though not psychopathologists, approached human emotion from a perspective which was inherently melancholic and steeped in pathos. Generally, the tragic sense of life has been prevalent among the existentialists, rather than the adaptive aspects of human psychology. Kierkegaard (1844/1957), with his work *The Concept of Dread*, was influential in shaping this predominant perspective.

Kierkegaard emphasised the vast diversity of thoughts and beliefs potentially available to each and every one of us. For Kierkegaard, however, most human beings resist the development of self-understanding, living in fear of intellectual freedom. This avoidance of the capacity to understand is said by Kierkegaard to be based on the fear, or 'dread', of the truth concerning the nature of existence, which is unbearable to all but the enlightened, those who have faced and accommodated to the actualities of existence following considerable self-disciplined introspection.

Heidegger and Sartre developed Kierkegaard's notion of dread, particularly in outlining its implications. Heidegger (1927) distinguished between 'authentic' and 'inauthentic' modes of being, either of which may be adopted by an individual, depending upon whether there is a need for denial of or receptivity to basic truth at any given time. During authentic being, we allow ourselves the freedom to realise that the range of thoughts, feelings and actions are infinite. Whatever subjective experiences and actions come into play, they are under the control (and, therefore, the responsibility) of oneself. Ways of construing, and therefore the scope of perception, are flexible and limitless, tending to be in a state of flux.

Heiddeger's concept of 'inauthenticity' and Sartre's (1943/1957) concept of 'bad faith' convey a particular perversity of human existence. Bad faith and inauthenticity arc the products of coping strategies to defend against the reality of existence, in which truth becomes under-represented in order that we may feel comfortable or secure. We may choose to ignore the knowledge that life is finite and that existence inevitably ends in death. We may choose the path of conformity of belief as a means of falsely reassuring ourselves that individual responsibility and self-determination is neither necessary nor accessible. The predominantly inauthentic individual is engaged in frequent self-evasiveness. This profoundly affects the scope of perceptual awareness and the degree of autonomy with which the individual is able to engage in decision-making in dealing with self and world.

The authentic individual has come to terms with his/her own ultimate fate, and the ambiguity of infinite possibility, by confronting meaninglessness and isolation. Spinelli attempts a comparison of authentic and inauthentic being:

> Rather than reacting as victims to the vicissitudes of being, we, as authentic beings, acknowledge our role in determining our actions, thoughts and beliefs, and thereby experience a stronger and fuller sense of integration, acceptance, openness and aliveness to the potentialities of being-in-the-world.
>
> In contrast, our thoughts and behaviour as inauthentic beings are marked by conventionality and conformity to the prevailing attitudes and morality of the culture that we reside in. As inauthentic beings, we respond to the experiences of life from a passive, reactive and ultimately unresponsible/irresponsible stance.

(Spinelli 1989: 109)

In some respects, inauthenticity resembles the position of external locus of control (Rotter 1966), but it is much wider than Rotter's concept, in incorporating limitations in the creative interpretation of self/world events rather than focusing on the more specific idea of the instrumentality of the individual.

Some writers who fit broadly under the existentialist umbrella, including Maslow (1968) and Rogers (1961), have pondered on the subjective nature of positive well-being, though the positive experiences of self-actualisation has not been fully explored as an emotional state. One notable exception is the self-actualising experience of heightened visual appreciation, which a number of art philosophers speak about.

The emotional state which is said to accompany aesthetic pleasure is termed 'aesthetic experience', a state which is marked by a distraction away from interoceptive stimulation so that exteroceptive perception is enhanced. Aesthetic experience is a meditative state, which enables the participant to enhance perceptual involvement by a reduction of self-awareness. This 'special' emotion is discussed more fully in Chapter 9.

There is little dialogue between existentialists and cognitive therapists. This is perhaps because each party has approached emotion from its own particular level. Existential considerations of emotionality encapsulate what is in essence a meta-construct of experience. Distress is viewed not from the point of view of the immediate psychological sequelae which emerge, but from that of the wider, more abstract, issues of being. Arguably, cognitive psychology, with its joint emphasis on thoughts, feeling and action plans, may go further than existentialism in constructing a science of being; cognitive techniques are often concerned with concretising the possibilities for predicted modes of existence by encouraging the patient to project into the future in a given set of circumstances.

This is the essence of Beck's (1963) 'vertical arrow' approach, whereby the subject traces the validity of present thoughts and feelings by laying bare their implications. The client is then challenged about the validity of these assumed implications. In doing so, various levels of cognitive operations are exposed, including automatic 'taken-for-granted' conjecture. If we compare the vertical-arrow method with the existential analysis of awareness of everyday being, we would suggest they both attempt to reflect a *Dasein-analysis*; each takes a cross-section of various levels of current psychological functioning, ranging from surface cognitions to assumptions of which the subject is barely aware, but which are nonetheless psychoactive.

Though the approach of cognitive therapy endorses the essence of the phenomenological method, it has failed to adopt the existential position. Heidegger's and Sartre's ideas on the fear and the futility of existence are theory-driven observations, and not sufficiently data-driven (i.e. not sufficiently borne out by observational evidence) to have impressed leading cognitive theorists so far. Though resistance to change during therapy may involve a reluctance in some clients to contemplate a broader potential repertoire of emotions, cognition and behaviours, not all distressed people present with doubts about life choices and the ethical dilemmas of their existence. Neither do they necessarily shy away from ambiguity and infinite possibility. In the clinical field, where patients complain of a diversity of experiential, emotional and ego-dystonic problems, there is a range of experience which goes beyond the preconceived subjective conditions to which Heidegger or Sartre felt human distress can be attributed. However, this apparent incompatibility may lie in the fact that the concepts of dread, bad faith and nausea were not designed as emotional concepts in the modern sense.

The concerns of the existentialists were wider than felt-states and cognition, and could feasibly be assumed to pertain to a broad-based implicational level underlying propositional self-statements, particularly concerning purposeful existence. Existential considerations may be of clinical value to cognitive therapy, but only if ambiguity of purpose and the infinity of psychological potential can be demonstrated as being intrinsically distressing. The area of 'dread' is relatively unexplored by cognitive therapists, but has a flavour which resembles the fear of ambiguity that many obsessional patients exhibit.

Cognitive therapists have tended to concentrate on surface cognitions, in the form of patients' verbal reports, and then infer deeper structures, such as core assumptions, after examining themes in the manifest verbal self-report. Generally speaking, cognitive psychopathologists have concentrated on analysing the linguistic patterns and evaluative perceptions of their patients, reflecting the immediacy of the concerns of distressed subjects and the underlying organisation of such preoccupation. However, some cognitive theorists have began to consider emotions as possessing organised structure, too, and the concept of affective or emotional schemata is beginning to gain popularity (see, for example, Beck *et al.* 1990; Safran and Greenberg 1991). However, the relationship between cognitive and emotional schemata is still unclear.

Rice and Greenberg (1984) recommend looking for key transition points in the presentation of patients during therapy, especially moments when sensations or thoughts change dramatically. They observe that sudden changes in the affect or content of self-report tend to occur during the course of an interview situation. These points are considered crucial, since they represent potential changes in direction of thought and feeling (and, hence, changes in schematic activation), forming the basis for making the subject aware of sources of fluctuation in state. Such changes in the flow of self-report may form a window for change, in that there is an opportunity for the therapist to highlight specific stages in the cognitive flow which usher in affective change, including the maladaptive states. How these variations in presentation are capitalised upon is dependent on the therapist's own style and skill, but, ironically, swings in mood during a clinical session and spontaneous self-modification of conversational content often go unnoticed during therapy.

Underlining this investment in spontaneous affective fluctuation, Greenberg and Safran (1987) postulate that authenticity of emotion occurs spontaneously in consciousness, but, subsequently, is rapidly obscured by social learning. The aim of their approach to therapy is to sharpen the client's discrimination between spontaneous and controlled emotions, and to focus their attention on the 'authentic' emotions. There is an assumption that these primary, fleeting emotions are important markers of psychoactive schemata.

THE NOTION OF FIXED EMOTIONAL TYPES

Psychophysiological theories of emotion

Many theories have taken on the task of locating the source of emotion. Emotional concepts are theory-driven, each theoretical position generating its own hypothesis about the origin and nature of emotional reactions. Typologies are in part determined by the hypothesised source of the emotional reaction, whether it has a somatic, social or self-referential basis. The search for emotional 'essence' in terms of discrete irreducible phenomena is futile, in real terms, if we adopt the view that emotionality involves an interaction of several modes of functioning.

The definition of emotion and the structuring of emotional theories are intrisically linked. For example, the traditionally established emotional vectors of anxiety and depression in clinical psychology and psychiatry have tended to stress the biological aspects of emotion, endorsing the classical approach. Classical theories view emotion ultimately as an internal state triggered by the release of biochemical substrates and neurophysiological or other somatic events.

Current theories of the 'drives' or 'dispositions' of emotion derive directly from the Greek humour theories, which postulated that emotion was a product of bodily fluids and arose by a process akin to internal combustion. Plato and Aristotle considered emotions to be base and without direction, over which active reason could exercise some control. Rational, self-initiated thought was a function of the immortal 'psyche' whereas passions were extensions of the soma. The Stoics regarded emotions as diseases similar to physical illness. The traditional clinical approach to emotion has, in the past, been essentially reductionist, both in theory and measurement.

In the 1950s and 1960s, there was a great deal of interest in physiological criteria which could be taken by physically unintrusive means, particularly as indices of anxiety. These measures included Galvanic Skin Response (minute changes in electrical skin conductance), EMG at various sites, ECG and EEG, and forearm bloodflow. Empirical attempts were made to describe physiological profiles specific to each of the emotions (Ax 1953). Lacey and Lacey (1958) hypothesised that a specific emotion would give rise to a corresponding psychophysiological profile, unique to that emotion and common to all subjects.

Unfortunately, attempts to identify strong correlations between physiological criteria and a specific emotion have not been successful. This is because the same psychophysiological criterion is often associated with a variety of opposing emotions. For example, the magnitude of skin conductance is similar during anxiety, surprise, embarrassment, shame and fear. Similarly, acceleration in respiration rate has been found at the outset of startle, anxiety, fear, surprise and relief (see, for example, O'Gorman 1973); anger can produce both an increase or decrease in diastolic blood pressure. Both quiet contentment and embarrassment can produce peripheral vasodilation. Divergence between various autonomic measures previously assumed to measure the same emotion is also common. Lader (1972) found consistently low correlations between bloodflow, heart-rate and skin conductance during anxiety. Obrist (1981) extensively discusses cardiac-somatic uncoupling (i.e. divergence between heart-rate and muscle activity). Such data help provide a rationale for the limited efficacy of biofeedback as a treatment method, particularly when used in the absence of other approaches.

The search for emotion-specific psychophysiological arousal criteria has largely been abandoned. Instead, such criteria have been accepted as general measures of 'activation' (see, for example, Neiss 1988), but are not differentiated sufficiently to account for specific qualities of consciousness. There is some justification for regarding arousal criteria as a measure of intensity of feeling, though it is now generally agreed that the quality and hedonic tone of feeling is not reflected by physiological amplitude. Furthermore, a subject's appraisal of interoceptive stimuli arising out of the same somatic activity is variable, depending on how the individual makes sense of a sensory event at the moment the sensations appear. For example, when patients are taught to tolerate and understand the effects of hyperventilation, the significance of the sensations diminishes and the response to the same amplitude of somatic output ceases to be one of alarm (Clark 1988).

Evolutionary theories and the classification of emotionality

Darwin's (1872) concept of evolution by natural selection had a profound influence on the biological sciences. One of the major implications of Darwin's model was that the characteristics of species reflected biological necessity. Within the emotional context, fear is seen by evolutionists to have distinct and sophisticated biological properties, which serve to enhance defence or escape and thereby protect the organism against physical harm. Modern emotional theories have linked basic emotions closely to current knowledge of the 'primitive' brain.

Fonberg (1986) states that emotional events relate to biological needs and constitute 'fuel for drives', and hence determine the negative and positive hedonic value of internal and external events. Fonberg considers that the evaluation of sensory input culminates in the amygdala, which assesses internal and external stimuli with respect to biological usefulness, with the survival utility being communicated to the organism in the form of hedonic tone. Survival-friendly objects and activities are imbued with pleasant characteristics, while objects and activities which pose a threat to the organism and to the species are felt as aversive and therefore elicit an avoidance reaction. Within the amygdaloid complex there is an excitatory dorso-medial part, which is thought to control apathy and sadness, and an inhibitory lateral part, related to joyfulness and liveliness, and it is in these areas that the link between stimulus and survival behaviour is said to be mediated, inhibiting behaviour towards biologically-detrimental stimuli and exciting approach behaviour to biologically-advantageous stimuli.

Izard (1972) is an exponent of the evolutionary approach to emotion and takes the view that anger, contempt, disgust, distress, fear, guilt, interest, joy and shame are the standard, universal human emotions. Izard considers these to be functionally linked to neural circuits and, therefore, to provide the species with a predetermined range or menu of emotional responses. Despite the 'hard-wired menu' of emotional options, humans, unlike lower organisms, are viewed as portraying considerable flexibility in the actual manifestations of emotional behaviour; excitation of the respective neural circuit is said to be influenced by experience, which determines both categorisation of the stimulus situation and the means of emotional expression. Gray (1982) also adopts the hard-wired hypothesis, but limits the fixed emotional types to rage, anxiety and joy.

In the hard-wired theoretical context, clinical anxiety is construed as the inappropriate triggering of the fight–flight response, in the absence of genuine threat. This position is compatible with cognitive theories of emotion, since the inappropriate elicitation of threat is viewed by Gilbert (1993) as the product of inaccurate appraisal of environmental cues. Gilbert suggests that there is an inbred tendency for humans to be over-inclusive in their appraisal of what is dangerous and that this in itself has survival value, on the assumption that it is 'better to be safe than sorry'. Gilbert proposes that neurotic patients have a relatively more sensitive alarm-trigger mechanism, but that the threshold above which it is provoked can be raised by the subject's reappraisal of what is dangerous. Post-traumatic stress disorder (PTSD) is a vivid example of a defensive psychological posture, and is defined by the prolongation of alarm, the onset of which is subsequent to a discrete traumatic experience. Viewing PTSD as the persevering excitation of the 'hard-wired' biological alarm system long after the eliciting threat has receded may prove a useful model within which the syndrome can be investigated. The crucial task is how to access the schema, which continually activates the alarm.

Both Gilbert (1993) and Gray (1987) extend Darwinian ideas to affective disorder, viewing depression as a natural, hard-wired response to excessive punishment and failure; when the environment is hostile and fails to provide reward, both authors postulate that it is adaptive in the natural state for an organism to possess a mechanism which diminishes expectations and inhibits exploratory behaviour; the organism consequently enters a phase of withdrawal and, so the theory goes, consequently retreats from an unproductive interaction with a threatening milieu. Depressive mood, therefore, is viewed as a mechanism by which the organism is temporarily extricated from risk, as part of a self-protective defence system. By contrast, Gilbert (1993) views hypomania as a mechanism by which outgoing and adventurous behaviour may be effected.

One of the main problems for the reductionist approaches to the classification of the human emotions is the glaring discrepancy in the scope and subtle variation of emotional states between the general public and some theoreticians; one may legitimately ask how Averill's (1975) 500 adjectives, reflecting the layman's nosology, can be reduced to a mere half a dozen or so theoretical emotional constructs. One explanation, provided by a theoretical adjunct to 'core' theories of emotion, is the simultaneous occurrence of two or more emotional types, which Scherer (1984) refers to as 'palette theories'.

An advocate of palette theory is Plutchick (1980), who proposes a psychoevolutionary model that identifies eight basic emotions: acceptance, anger, anticipation, disgust, joy, fear, surprise and sadness. The complexity of emotions recognised in human beings are, according to Plutchick, combinations of these basic, primary emotions; for example, pride is a mix of anger and joy. Plutchick draws an analogy between emotion mixes and colour mixtures. All the colours of the spectrum can be obtained by combining a limited number of primaries. From a clinical point of view, Plutchick's model would suggest that some emotions are incompatible while others might more readily blend together and transform one another. For example, sadness and joy could not be expressed at the same time, whereas anger and disgust could be felt simultaneously as resentment or revulsion.

Plutchick defines emotion as a complex process with neurophysiological, neuromuscular and subjective aspects. Emotion is hypothesised as arising out of a series of biologically-programmed interoceptive cues. Plutchick (1980) states that innately programmed chemical activity produces patterned facial and bodily activities and that feedback from these activities is transformed into conscious form, resulting in a discrete fundamental emotion. According to Plutchick, molecular events transform into psychological events via neuromuscular activity. The model implies a special type of motor schema which influences affective schemas. That apart, there may be some value in attempting a classification of irreducible feeling states as components of emotional response. A growing amount of research has been devoted recently to a nosology of 'basic' feeling states. A valuable contribution that hard-wired theories make to subjective psychology may turn out to be the addressing of the issue of classification of feeling. We simply do not know what the discrete entities of feeling are, nor whether it is legitimate to regard feelings as multidimensional affect.

Whichever emotional types are assumed to constitute the clutch of basic emotions, palette theorists consider that it is rare that a singular, 'core' emotion will be present in consciousness in normal everyday existence. The presence of simultaneous emotions raises an interesting issue: if two emotions can be present in consciousness at any given moment, will the subject experience both, in their original form, or will the emotions interact to form a singular, more elaborate emotion, which is qualitatively different from either of its constituents? Opinion among palette theorists is divided; Averill (1975) suggests that the primary emotions rarely or never exist as solitary states, but, rather, occur in combinations which metamorphose, resulting in an almost infinite variety of subtle emotional hues and blends. Plutchick (1962) and Ekman (1982) suggest that emotions may co-exist simultaneously, but each retains its original properties.

It is not clear to what degree Beck et al. (1990) regard affective schemata as personalised, nor whether they take the view that affective schemas are infinitely variable. There is, therefore, much scope for postulating the nature of affective organisation, and for consideration of whether affective schemata are reoccurring 'palettes' of fixed combinations of feeling unique to each individual. This issue may have implications for Beck's notion of affective schemas, the properties and organisation of which remain largely undocumented. Currently, we do not know whether affective schema consist of palettes of feeling states which co-vary in a personalised manner, nor whether there are fixed relationships between certain feeling states.

The above proposal begs the question of whether the components of an emotional configuration can be teased out. Watts (1992) provides an anecdotal clinical example of the extrication of two feeling states that are habitually activated simultaneously. He points out that arachnophobics react to spiders with a mixture of fear and disgust. Following numerous observations, involving several patients, Watts observed that live spiders elicit a roughly equal intensity of the two emotions. By contrast, when exposed to dead spiders, the emotional response was different. Dead spiders elicit almost the same intensity of disgust as live ones, but noticeably less fear. For emotional-schema theorists, the quantitative differentiation of emotionality illustrates the fluidity of affective schemata accorded by changes in the identifying of the spider as 'dead' or 'alive'. Presumably, the identification is accompanied by a reorientation of instrumental schemas and schemas relating to control and self-efficacy in the changed situation, in addition to the selective activation of feeling states on the affective palette.

There have been other attempts to outline fixed patterns of affective organisation when more than one identifiable feeling is involved. For example, Tyrer (1982) considers irritability to be a symptom of anxiety. However, Snaith and Taylor (1985), using the Irritability, Depression and Anxiety Scale (IDAS), concluded that irritability is present in all types of psychological disturbance. Snaith and Taylor administered the scale repeatedly to several patients and were able to examine the co-variance of the two states longitudinally across patients.

Theories of emotion as social communication

Social psychologists stress that the crucial element in emotion lies in its expression – emotion is not a reflection of an internal state, but a reflection of a perceiving and communicating self. Emotion would hence be seen as a vehicle for manipulating or changing a course of interaction, of drawing attention, or of making an impression by acting out an action-disposition. In this case, the clinician should be looking for the role that a played emotion implies. Emotion as a behaviour has a prospective, feed-forward function, so that a person adopts a certain role not because of events, but *in order to elicit them*. This idea of emotion reverses the conventional cognitive or evolutionary model of emotions as products, and suggests that an emotion may be progressively constituted as the person acts it out.

Darwin's (1872) theory was not totally preoccupied with morphology, since Darwin also postulated that emotional responsivity has a role in regulating social interaction, by providing participants with visible cues of each other's internal state. Darwin saw clear advantages to the gregariousness of many of the higher species, and viewed social behaviour as an attribute with a clear survival function, particularly in fostering activities in which members of a species could co-operate as a group. Some predators hunt in packs, some members of the pack driving their quarry towards other members lying in waiting. In man, the formation of social groups into communities permitted the division of labour, so that some individual members specialised in one activity, while others specialised in another, to the mutual benefit of the group as a whole. Darwin acknowledged the fact that human groups develop their own rules, in terms of specific cultures and traditions, and saw the evolution of cultural phenomena as also subject to the laws of survival of the fittest. Hence, those groups and societies with the best survival-oriented cultures flourish, while others fail to compete and are either wiped out or capitulate to the fitter culture. For humans to function as a group, transmission of information between individual group members is essential and Darwin viewed emotion as a means of communication, by prompting visible, nonverbal changes. Darwin cited his comparative studies as evidence of how current emotional expression had derived from lower animal forms. This anthropological theme has since been popularised by Desmond Morris *et al.* (1979). The interpretation of some facial expression – e.g. as friendly or unfriendly – is considered innate.

An enigmatic example of a communicated emotional response, which is of considerable theoretical interest, is blushing. Blushing is an involuntary reflex causing vasodilation in the cheeks. It is elicited exclusively by social stimuli, and accompanied by thoughts of shame and embarrassment (Shean *et al.* 1992). Darwin (1872) explained it as the 'leaking' or signalling of an emotional condition to others around oneself. He noted that attempts to control it only worsened the blushing. Edelmann (1987), a psychophysiologist, hypothesised that blushing serves the purpose of alerting the self to one's embarrassment. But it is difficult to see the 'function' of publicising disgrace, or how the physiological components of blushing relate functionally to subjective components.

Certainly, not all somatic output is independent of emotional subjective activity. Affective and motor indices taken from highly specific sites are highly correlated with qualitative aspects of emotion, and that is particularly true of striate muscle activity involved in facial, nonverbal, social communication; motor activity, particularly facial expression, has been consistently identified with specific emotional states. *Fear*, for example, involves forceful blinking, frowning, stooping and hunching the shoulders protectively. *Surprise* involves widening of the eyes, reduction of muscle tone and momentary lack of mobility. *Anger* involves a fixed stare, widened eyes, contracted eyebrows, muscle tension and clenched fists. *Sadness* involves turning down of the mouth, lowered muscle tone and downcast eyes. These expressions seem consistent across cultures (Ekman 1982).

Data which has been interpreted as unambiguous evidence for fixed emotional types is provided from the work of Ekman and Oster (1979), who have studied recognition of facial expression across cultures, both eastern, western and aboriginal. Ekman, like Izard, postulates a core affect programme which is genetically based and closely associated with the innervation of the face. For Ekman, culture may determine the kind of situations that elicit emotion and the coping response to them, but the *expression* of emotion is a constant. Whereas some investigators, such as Birdwhistel (1970), challenge the idea of universal expressions, there is wide support for the position of Ekman (1984), who found cross-cultural consistency in facial expressions of strong emotions, despite wide cultural variability in other demonstrative emotional signals, such as loudness of voice, bodily contact and mobility, and hand gestures.

COMMUNICATIVE FACIAL EXPRESSION AS A DETERMINANT OF EMOTION

In line with Plutchick's (1980) hypothesis that proprioceptive cues arising from the facial musculature are independant variables of felt emotion, strategies for emotional manipulation based on the musculature of facial expression have been attempted. Laird and Eckman have sought directly to influence mood through manipulating facial expression. Laird *et al.* (1982) asked experimental subjects to frown or smile for around ten minutes' duration and noted corresponding changes on mood scales taken immediately after, using the Adjective Mood Scale. A similar finding was reported by Riskind (1983), who, in addition to facial expression, manipulated body position consistent with happiness or sadness (chest expanded with body upright and erect *versus* neck bowed, body stooped and slumped). In a recent study and review, Levenson *et al.* (1990) instructed subjects to mimic facially the emotions of disgust, fear, happiness, sadness and surprise. They found that directed facial expression produces significant levels of the respective emotions. Some people enacting the emotion reported experiencing an affective state to an extent normally associated with their undirected expression.

Levenson *et al.* (1990) suggest they have found a way to induce emotions physiologically, though they are uncertain of the mechanisms. They suggest four separate psychophysiological models. The first model states that voluntary facial configurations trigger signals from the motor cortex to the autonomic system. The second model posits a central pattern detector which scans efferent outflow and then activates an affect programme. The third model postulates that afferent feedback from facial contractions creates emotion. And the fourth model states that the connection between facial expression and emotionally-specific autonomic activity is socially learned.

The limitations of the facial-feedback studies are that, in general, the emotional experiences generated by voluntary contraction are not the same as those generated in real life. The subjects used in the studies were selected on a *priori* grounds for their ability to produce convincing facial expressions, and many were trained actors. Another methodological problem is that in order to manipulate facial musculature, subjects may have achieved the required expression by 'thinking themselves into the role'; therefore, other cognitive factors could be involved in following instructions to pull a face. As a consequence, mood change could have preceded the change in facial expression, rather than being the product of it. The methodological problem is not insurmountable: a procedure similar to that of Gilligan and Bower (1984) could be used, in which hypnotically-induced amnesia could be employed to discontinue the stream of thought and emotion, at the point at which the appropriate facial expression was achieved. The effect of the expression on subsequent emotion could then be documented.

Even though there may be consistency across societies, anthropologists have noted that social situations within cultures elicit different emotions, and some have proposed that social context may be the determining factor in the labelling of an affective state. As Franks and McCarthy put it:

> There may be universal emotions (e.g. anger) but this in no way undermines the arguments that emotions are cultural and historical ways of experiencing and acting capable of considerable variation in both what is felt and in the meaning of what is felt.

> (Franks and McCarthy 1989)

The interpersonal argument is that it is purely interpersonal factors, such as social distance or adopted roles, that determine the emotion expressed. Physiological factors are either uniform or at best the tail end of the emotional act. The social theorists move away from what Averill (1975) termed the 'reifying tendencies' of emotion and instead consider it to be as an ecological 'process'. There is no emotion without context, since one has to be emotional about something. Only when percepts are invested with meaning can an emotion occur.

In this respect, the theory of emotion put forward by Ortony *et al.* (1988) deserves a mention. This is a theory which goes some way to explain the source of the variability of emotionality, based on the perspective of appraisal or intention- ality of the subject. The authors feel that, though cognitive appraisal is central to the formation of emotional experience, the systematic differentiation of cognitive appraisal has not been sufficiently outlined. Ortony *et al.* suggest that emotional variability is based on the focus of appraisal of the individual at any given moment, and that there are three broad areas of appraisal within which emotionality occurs, namely, appraisal pertaining to objects, events and agents. Objects refer to distal stimuli representing concrete objects, which impinge on the subject's awareness; events refer to the subjective assessment of what has happened; agents refer to the processes and things which are construed to be of causal significance, and therefore the focus on agents reflects the attributional rationale which the subject attaches to an object or event. This model offers a means by which emotions can be differen- tiated and the examples of differentiation provided by Ortony *et al.* make it obvious that emotional quality is determined by the subject's reference point, that is, whether the appraisal is of objects, events or the source of their instrumentality (agents).

Ortony *et al.* (1988) reject the current attempts at emotional typology, since the latter mistakenly concentrate on emotion as subjective atmosphere alone, while ignoring the subject matter around which the emotion arises. Emotions only exist in conscious awareness and Ortony *et al.*'s model is couched in the context of what one is aware of, rather than a vacuous state. For example, the evaluative reaction to an event produces a different emotional form depending on assessment of the event as good or bad, and the source of instrumentality. Reaction to one's own desirable actions may result in the emotion of pride, while the desirable actions of others result in the emotion of admiration. Conversely, disapproval of one's own undesirable actions results in guilt and shame, while reaction to undesirable, disapproved-of actions attributed to others results in reproach.

Ortony *et al.*'s (1988) theory places emotionality in a social context, and illustrates mechanisms of social perspective which differentiate emotional quality on the basis of perceived repercussions of events for 'myself' or 'other person'. If I am displeased about an event that is to someone else's advantage, I am likely to feel resentment. On the other hand, if I am displeased about an event that is to someone else's disadvantage, I am likely to feel sorrow and sympathy. Pleasure at the misfortune of another will manifest as gloating, while pleasure at a good-fortune event for the other person will lead to a 'happy-for' emotion.

Ortony *et al.* (1988) have constructed a theory which integrates evaluative perspectives tied to the subject's social world, and incorporates attributional style into its axiomatic structure. Attribution and the 'I' versus 'others' perspective are important new areas in delusional thinking. Later in this chapter, we will refer to the emotional atmosphere that immediately precedes delusion-formation, which appears to precede firm attributional judgements. During this phase, sometimes referred to as a delusional mood or atmosphere, there is often considerable indecision and a failure to generate any firmly-held evaluative judgements, until the moment when the delusion emerges into consciousness. Before discussing this state further, we now turn to the issue of emotional creativity.

Creative emotional expression

Some therapists regard facial expression as an important concomitant of emotional change. There is a growing eclectic tendency in the cognitive movement to move away from verbal to experientially-broader methodologies. This is because the emotions engage several modes, or schema. Mahoney (1991), in a recent key founder's address, said he looked forward to cognitivists dealing less with a bodiless head and more with therapies which use the body. Treatment approaches which engage nonverbal aspects of emotion, such as body language and the motor components of emotional expression, are becoming more popular and have always had a place in therapy techniques.

Lusebrink (1992), in a recent article on expressive therapies, proposed that all therapies occupy points on three continua. She suggests that a systems approach allows the therapies to be organised and divided along dimensions in accordance with three hierarchical levels: kinesthetic/sensory, perceptual/affective, and cognitive/symbolic. She proposes that certain activities induce emotionally potent proprioceptive and kinesthetic feedback, such as relaxation, or the immersion in unpredictable motor activities, such as dance therapy or movement improvisation. The perceptual-affective level may be addressed through specific evocative images produced by art therapy and imagination. The cognitive-symbolic level emphasises the analytical, logical and reality-directed aspects of information processing. (This is the level most 'talking' therapies purport to engage.) Lusebrink sees clients as over- or under-distanced to these modalities, and the mode of therapy may need to be chosen to compensate for these needs. She suggests that an important aspect of any level of therapy is for the client to be creative at that level. Creativity is viewed as lying somewhere between inhibited and impulsive expressions.

This notion of creativity is not dwelt on by traditional cognitive therapy, in which procedures are very seldom spontaneous and tend on the whole to be formalised, controlled and principally stress conformity to a rational protocol. The use of the imagination is employed in cognitive therapy, but largely as a means of revealing barely conscious assumptions, particularly in time-projection exploratory 'vertical arrow' techniques. The existential notion of 'infinite possibility' mentioned above, appears more aligned to creative processes and discovery and treats imagination as an equal part of experience.

EMOTIONALITY SURROUNDING DELUSION-FORMATION

One of the commonest features of patients with severe mental health problems is the formation of erroneous, bizarre beliefs, which are held with conviction in the face of overwhelming objective evidence to the contrary. Many patients act on their delusional beliefs and, since behaviour change is based on unannounced and false propositional self-statements, the resulting actions appear unpredictable and threatening to the uninformed observer, so that the patient often feels misunderstood and socially alienated. Not surprisingly, social rejection has a detrimental effect on the overall quality of a patient's life.

The nature of delusional thinking has been considered from a variety of perspectives, including attentional bias towards information confirming the delusion and attentional shift away from disconfirmatory evidence (Bullen and Hemsley 1987); distorted attributional style (Candido and Romney 1990); poor problem-solving performance and diminished hypothesis-testing ability (Garety et al. 1991). It is not established whether such dysfunctional characteristics are primary or secondary (i.e. whether they have an effect in generating a delusion or form the product of the delusion). The issue may prove to be less important than consideration of how these dysfuctional processes maintain the delusion once it is incorporated into the flow of thinking.

An area which is ripe for investigation is the nature and role of emotion during and following delusion-formation. We have seen in Chapter 2 that affect influences the content of thinking. Since delusional beliefs are propositional thoughts, it is legitimate to search for links between emotion and delusions. There are grounds for regarding deluded thinking as a product of an underlying emotional dysfunction. Delusional thinking is typically of sudden onset, with primary delusion beliefs flooding suddenly into consciousness. Secondary elaboration of delusional belief, based on extensions to the original premise, commonly follows. The spontaneous 'out-of-the blue' occurrence of primary delusions is inexplicable, both in form and content. The content is particularly abstruse when it is unrelated to any overvalued ideas or pre-morbid concerns of the patient. Though the onset of delusional thinking is sudden, characteristic emotional changes are widely acknowledged prior to delusion-formation. These changes consist of abnormal feeling states, often accompanied by a reduction in intense propositional thinking, until the point at which the delusion crystallises.

Delusional ideas are usually preceded by marked vigilance, perplexity and suspicion. This evaluative mode is typically shrouded by an atmosphere of distrust and unpredictability. The patient becomes extremely guarded and is preoccupied with the impression that there is something undefinably strange or sinister about the surrounding world and, because of this, he or she takes on a defensive disposition. In the words of Berner, this experience is

> characterised by the failure to retain the space between perceived facts and what is behind them. The background loses its neutrality, and the patient becomes like an anxious child walking through a wood. Nothing is evident and natural any more. The particularity of this suspicion is that the patient is not struck by what people do or say but what they don't do or say. This process develops into an overall change of the perception of the entire outside world and causes the patient to query his own existence.

> (Berner 1991)

Psychopathologists are divided over what this experience comprises. Some prefer to view it primarily as a type of mood disorder.

This position is characteristic of German phenomenologists, who, in view of their emphasis on the affective component, describe the state as 'delusional mood' (Jaspers 1963). The term is less popular with English-speaking psychiatrists, who consider the reference to a primary mood state as misleading, since there is an inherent assumption that perceptual and evaluative changes are secondary to the mood change. To avoid this assumption, the term 'delusional atmosphere' is preferred (Berner 1991). The term 'atmosphere' should not be taken to refer to exteroceptive events; it refers to the subjective atmosphere in which external events are construed.

It is after exposure to the above subjective conditions that delusions are said to arise. The experience of delusional atmosphere may last for several weeks or months, during which time the patient is engaged in a constant search for the meaning behind the intuitive sense of foreboding and insecurity. Delusional beliefs characteristically enter consciousness spontaneously as sudden, immediate cognitions. Though the content of the delusion is false, the belief is experienced as a remarkable insight, which is received with considerable relief and tension reduction. Suddenly, the patient feels that the world has become comprehensible once more. Delusional perceptions are, as Mellor puts it:

> usually preceded by a state of delusional atmosphere, which is an extremely unpleasant experience, characterised by uncertainty, anxiety, depression and perplexity. Familiar objects in the environment threaten but do not concede new

meanings. Suddenly, within this terrifying world, one perception stands out, because it has meaning that explains the strange experiences. This is the delusion, and with it comes a remarkable improvement in the patient's level of distress. The delusional atmosphere diminishes and the familiar meanings of other objects are no longer in doubt.

(Mellor 1991)

SUMMARY

In this chapter, we have attempted to outline some of the major approaches to a descriptive psychology of the emotions. There is no single, generally accepted nosology of the emotions, though a differentiation between 'core' and other emotional states is both popular and gaining appeal with some, but not all, empirical psychologists. It has been argued that recent attempts to tie basic emotions to fixed neurological structures are given support by the anthropological observation that there is an underlying fixedness in categories of emotional expression across diverse cultures. There is an assumption that uniformity of types of emotional expression implies uniformity of brain structures and a degree of neuroanatomic localisation of each basic emotion.

A competent model of emotion needs to be robust enough to incorporate variability due to attribution or set, subtlety of range of emotion, and emotions which accompany meaninglessness and excessive felt-meaning, particularly in psychotic breakdown. Though cognitive theories have made inroads into anxiety and mild–moderate depression, the emotionality surrounding the genesis of delusions has not been fully integrated into a comprehensive cognitive model.

Chapter 4

Panic disorder as a clinical entity

PANIC DISORDER AS A UNIQUE CATEGORY

Panic disorder is a term used to describe a sudden, apparently unprovoked, bout of intense fear, which is, according to DSM III, qualitatively distinct from the concept of anxiety. Panic is defined in DSM III(R) (1987) as a sudden rush of fear or impending doom, accompanied by four or more of the following: dyspnoea, palpitations, chest pain or discomfort, choking or smothering sensations, dizziness or unsteadiness, feelings of unreality, paresthesias, hot and cold flushes, sweating, faintness, trembling, a fear of dying, and fear of going mad or losing control. Barlow and Craske (1988) studied a group of forty-one agoraphobic subjects, all of whom exhibited panic disorder, in order to establish the prevalence of each of the above symptoms. The most common were palpitations (found in 98 per cent of the sample), dizziness (95 per cent), sweating (93 per cent), dyspnoea (90 per cent), and fear of going crazy or losing control (90 per cent). Barlow also asked his subjects to rate the intensity with which each of the DSM III(R) symptoms were felt, as a means of determining the degree of distress emanating from them. The four most prominently felt symptoms were palpitations, fear of dying, dizziness and trembling, in that order.

The distinction between a generalised anxiety state and panic in the DSM III implies that the difference between the two is qualitative rather than simply quantitative, otherwise there would be no reason to go beyond the diagnosis 'severe generalised anxiety disorder'. There is considerable clinical evidence to support the notion that panic is distinct from anxiety. One particularly convincing strand of evidence is that patients who have both disorders discriminate clearly between them. At a given moment in time, they are able to report quantitative changes in each, which are divergent.

Waddel *et al*. (1984) observed three subjects who exhibited both chronic anxiety and panic while they were under treatment. The treatment consisted of relaxation training and cognitive therapy, the effects of which were measured by self-monitoring over a period of several weeks. The self-rating measures included the recording of generalised, background anxiety, and sudden bouts of panic. Their results showed that the subjective measures for anxiety and panic did not co-vary, particularly in two of the three subjects; while chronic background anxiety diminished in response to the cognitive-behavioural treatment, panic attacks occurred with the same frequency and intensity.

It has been suggested by Clark (1988) and Hibbert (1984b) that a major distinguishing feature between the two states is the content of thought during an attack. Anxious patients are likely to become preoccupied with their inability to overcome the distress and to dread becoming conspicuous by seeming odd and bizarre in a social context. They feel they will make fools of themselves and be rejected by others, or lose face. The content of negative expectancy is based on humiliation and embarrassment. Thinking during panic disorder, however, is said to take a different course, involving despair oriented around physical or psychological welfare, so that the panic patient fears death, especially from heart attack or suffocation, or, alternatively, becomes convinced that the experience will lead to madness or dementia.

Beck (1988) also distinguishes panic from anxiety in cognitive terms; panic is particularly marked by the complete absence of moderating, reflective activity, so that negative, catastrophic assumptions, such as those mentioned above, roll on uncontrollably and are unchallenged by counterbelief. For Beck, a panic attack is characterised by the inability to overview internal events and put them in perspective. For example, placing attacks in the context of previous distressing episodes which ended innocuously is characteristic of some anxiety states, but not of panic disorder.

SELF-BODY RELATIONS DURING PANIC

There is some evidence from physiological studies that panic disorder is characterised by hyperventilation to a greater degree than generalised anxiety. Among others, Hibbert (1986) has reported low blood carbon dioxide typical of hyperventilation during naturally-occurring panic attacks. Consistent with the above, Rapee (1985) measured resting heart- and respiration-rate (during subjectively 'safe' periods) in both generalised anxiety and panic patients. Rapee found that the latter had a significantly higher heart-rate and a significantly greater tendency to overbreathe than the anxiety patients, during corresponding intervals of subjective safety. He concluded that panic patients may be vulnerable to further exacerbation of panic when exposed to even minor environmental stressors, because baseline blood carbon dioxide is already abnormally low, so that any further carbon dioxide diminution due to accelerated respiration cannot be accommodated.

We have discussed, in Chapter 3, the imperfect relationship between physiological measures and distress. The assumption that raised arousal criteria are an essential prerequisite of panic is open to question; some patients, for example, have indicated that they are experiencing a full-blown panic attack when their internal physiological conditions, measured as heart-rate, reflect those of baseline and non-panicking controls (Taylor *et al.* 1986). Furthermore, neither hyperventilation *per se* nor the lowering of blood carbon dioxide by artificial means inevitably lead to panic.

Rapee (1986) observed a series of twenty panic patients during conditions of guided hyperventilation, i.e. during a period in which the subjects were instructed to hyperventilate intentionally. Though the majority of subjects experienced a sufficient range of somatic symptoms to match DSM III criteria, and despite the fact that the majority identified the symptoms as similar to a naturally-occurring panic, not one of Rapee's subjects reported an actual panic attack. Some subjects provided the rationale that panic did not occur because they felt safe within the confines of the clinical situation and because they were able to link the occurrence of the abnormal somatic sensations with the hyperventilation itself.

Interestingly, when non-clinical subjects are asked to hyperventilate, some claim enjoyment of the subjective consequences (Clark 1988). A broad conclusion stemming from these observations is that psychophysiology alone is a poor marker of the panic experience, but that panic is characterised by an overly dramatic, calamitous interpretation of such somatic changes.

COGNITION AND PANIC

Inconsistencies in psychophysiological output across patients during panic have lent considerable support to the hypothesis that aberrant psychophysiology *per se* is not the determinant of panic (Beck 1988), a conclusion which has shifted the attention of some clinicians onto the role of cognitive mechanisms in precipitating the disorder. This line of thinking is very much in keeping with the phenomeno-logical premise that a stimulus event (whether it be distal or interoceptive) has no intrinsic meaning, but is given psychological significance by the way in which it is interpreted. A popular view among cognitivists is that interoceptive stimuli arising from somatic sensations of arousal are perceived by the patient as being of over-inflated significance, so that such sensations are interpreted as signals of irreparable and irreversible morbidity (Barlow and Craske 1988). A more radical view is that physiological symptoms are mere artefacts of the panic experience, though by definition, the DSM III classification of panic does not uphold this view, since physiological symptoms make up a considerable part of the diagnostic picture.

'Normal panic' in the general population

In a study of the non-clinical population, Norton *et al.* (1986) found a high incidence of panic experiences according to DSM III qualitative criteria, apart from frequency of attacks. According to Norton *et al.*, 35 per cent of the normal population have experienced one or more panic attacks during the previous twelve months. Many authors view panic as a 'fear of fear' phenomenon; the first attack is considered to be important in generating anticipatory fears of further attacks and therefore the onset of panic symptoms are viewed as significant in providing material which will preoccupy the subject, changing self-image to that of a vulnerable person, prone to difficult experiences for which the subject envisages poor coping skills. Yet epidemiological survey data illustrate that not all individuals experiencing an initial attack will go on to develop further attacks. Therefore, some individuals escape the DSM III diagnosis by virtue of their subsequent ability to cope.

If there are differences between once-only or low-frequency panickers and those who fit DSM III criteria, it is pertinent to ask what those differences are. Are the differences based on frequency alone? It would appear that there are qualitative differences between non-clinical panickers and those fitting DSM III: Norton *et al.* (1986) compared the ratings of symptom severity with those explored by Barlow and Craske (1988). They observed that, in Barlow and Craske's sample of clinical panic, the so-called 'fears' symptom (fear of going mad or losing control) was ranked highest in terms of severity, while it was ranked sixth by their own sample of less-frequent, non-clinical panic subjects.

It may be productive to investigate the differences between clinical and non-clinical panic subjects further. When one considers that panic is present at low frequency in at least one-third of the normal population, it is a matter of considerable speculation what differences are to be found between 'normal' and 'pathogenic' panic. 'Survivors' of panic experiences may be utilising coping skills which multiple-attack patients could potentially acquire.

In one of his earlier influential works, Beck (1976) illuminated a common strategic problem with which clinicians are faced. When agoraphobics with panic attacks were asked which specific consequences they feared most in the situations they most dreaded, Beck drew a self-limited response containing little insight: the typical reply from his patients was that venturing out into the crowded streets, onto public transport, etc., was viewed with apprehension because panic attacks had been experienced there on prior occasions. Further, the first attack was described typically as coming 'out of the blue'. Such a dearth of information volunteered spontaneously from panic patients is commonplace and may explain why earlier writers have viewed panic attacks as being 'free-floating', or perhaps originating from the patient's state of physical health.

Beck, however, took the important step of training his patients in self-observation; they were urged to note both the sensations they experienced in anxiety-provoking situations, and the subsequent thoughts arising out of such awareness. Though he could not ascertain clearly from retrospective accounts the source of the first attack, Beck was impressed by the highly-systematic thought processes exhibited by his patients. Specific fears which correspond to the DSM III criteria of panic (the symptom profile was created four years later) were explicable in terms of the situation most feared. For example, Beck found that fear of enclosed spaces was associated with fears of suffocation; crowded streets and public transport were construed as danger situations because of potential accidents which could lead to fatality; bridges were associated with fears of falling.

Despite the importance of attribution and expectancy, the presence of low blood CO_2 and raised heart-rate in the majority of cases of panic disorder is typical and therefore the obligation to consider the role of bodily change in panic disorder is unavoidable. The question to be raised is not whether physiological change is usually present, but what status such change has in the genesis of the disorder. Physiological changes have been viewed variously as an additional symptom, the cause, or a major prompt to cognitions of catastrophisation; the latter implies that physical sensations arising out of hyperventilation, for instance, interact with cognitive activity.

If physiological shift is important in generating alarm in panic-disorder patients by exciting anticipation of a breakdown in physical well-being or survival, it is of considerable importance to ascertain how the physiological change excites the negative cognition. An hypothesis which has immediate appeal is that the sensations produced by raised physiology are in themselves an intrinsic source of alarm. For example, the heaving of the chest as the lungs inhale and expel air at an unusually high frequency might generate physical discomfort; or the pounding of the heart as the ventricles are flooded with and discharge blood may feel alien to the beholder. Interestingly, though the interoceptive sensations produced by the somatic shift may have a role in generating distress, distress is also generated in some patients when physiological change is *perceived* to have occurred in the absence of any actual changes in internal sensation.

Ehlers *et al.* (1986) linked twenty-five panic patients to ECG and fed back to individual subjects the actual cardiac output and, at a different stage of the experiment, a fictitious feedback of inflated output. As a group, the patients reacted detrimentally to the fictitiously inflated heart-rate feedback by becoming anxious, as measured by further heart-rate, systolic blood pressure and subjective criteria, a pattern not shared by matched, non-anxious controls, who were unmoved by the false feedback. The readiness to interpret false feedback as valid is possibly worth investigating further in the opposite direction, i.e. the exposure to benign false feedback in the presence of elevated arousal criteria, in order to investigate the relative influence of perceived arousal level to two contradictory sources of biological information, namely, interoceptive stimuli versus exteroceptive false feedback.

Differentiating between over-reaction to somatic discomfort on the one hand, and fears of ill-health in the absence of somatic cues on the other, is not without implications regarding clinical management. While there may be an element of hypochondriasis in both, panic based on fluctuation in respiration-rate, feelings of faintness or palpitations, trembling, etc., can be viewed as having more of a phobic component. For example, Eysenck (1968) has argued that in subjects who exhibit anxiety frequently, with somatic sequelae, such interoceptive cues quickly become associated with aversive experience and may become conditioned stimuli upon which further conditioned fear (and, subsequently, more intense interoceptive cues) are based.

An implication of the classical conditioning model is the prediction that repeated exposure to interoceptive cues, in the absence of a fearful situation, would lead to extinction. With this aim in mind, somatic sensations (the CS) have been elicited by the introduction of lactate infusion (Bonn *et al.* 1973) and carbon dioxide inhalation (Van den Hout 1988). In the latter study, both patients and non-patient controls were administered three sessions of air inhalation and six sessions of inhalation of a gaseous mix, the combination of which was 35 per cent CO_2, 65 per cent O_2. Each session consisted of ten inhalations. It is established that a single deep inhalation of a combination of the gases used provokes rapid respiration. Subjects were required to rate levels of anxiety after each inhalation on a scale of 1–100, in the absence of any cognitive intervention. The control subjects (N=8) remained fairly calm throughout, with only minor anxiety reactions to the introduction of the abnormal gaseous mixes. Panic-prone subjects (N=14) showed a marked anxiety reaction to raised carbon dioxide, particularly when raised carbon dioxide was not introduced in the initial sessions but following exposure to three sessions of air only. The most significant finding of the study was that the patient group demonstrated considerable habituation to the abnormal gaseous exposure. On the sixth consecutive exposure session, they were exhibiting anxiety decrements to around 25 per cent of the peak rating, to levels approaching that of the controls.

Panic and hypochondriasis

The diagnosis of hypochondriasis is given when there is a lasting preoccupation with a pathological process within one's own body in the absence of evidence to support that view and despite medical reassurance. It is often argued that hypochondriasis is a specific form of obsessional rumination, since it is intrusive, inappropriate, repetitive and perseverative. Given the panic-disorder patient's preoccupation with acute illness, is it feasible to conceptualise the fear of loss of control symptoms of panic disorder as an obsessional trait? It could be argued, for example, that panic disorder is the product of the superimposition of generalised anxiety and obsessional rumination; given the existence of these two disorders within the traditional framework of descriptive psychopathology, the need for a third category (of panic disorder) may add nothing new. After all, the coexistence of two states or diagnostic entities does not pose any particular difficulty nosologically, and is dealt with in other areas of psychopathology by the concept of 'overlay'. Hypochondriacal rumination has been suggested as setting the conditions for interoceptive over-attentiveness. However, it is questionable whether such cognitive activity precedes nocturnal panics.

Fears of ill-health which arise in the absence of somatic sensation differ from somatically-cued worry, since they are not necessarily based on interoceptive data. Salkovskis (1988) reflects that, phenomenologically, there is a great deal of similarity between panic disorder and hypochondriasis, in that in both there is excessive concern given to the breakdown of physical well-being. However, he draws a possible distinction between the two in that in hypochondriasis, as opposed to panic, the nature of the perceived pathogenic process is detached from immediacy. In hypochondriasis, the supposed disease often has an insidious course and is considered by the patient to require lengthy and thorough diagnostic investigation to locate its source. By contrast, panic is characterised by a sense of acute urgency, and the supposed pathological process is construed to lead to imminent deterioration, and perhaps fatality, within seconds or minutes; the subjects feel their survival is hanging in the balance at that very moment of distress and immediate assistance is felt to be imperative. An example cited by Salkovskis is that whereas the experience of dizziness might typically be interpreted as evidence of the development of a brain tumour by a hypochondriac, the same symptom would more likely be interpreted as the onset of a heart attack by a panic-prone patient. Alternatively, it could be argued that panic disorder is a particular form of hypochondriacal rumination, which is distinguished from other forms of hypochondriasis by the diseases contemplated, those contemplated in panic disorder being diseases in which manifestation is acute and the effects more immediately debilitating.

SOME COMPLEX PRESENTATIONS OF PANIC DISORDER

Relaxation-induced panic

Though most authors describe elevation of psychophysiological arousal as being a major prompt of panic attacks in prone individuals, there do appear to be apparent paradoxes in this respect. While taking physiological measures from patients undergoing relaxation training, Cohen *et al.* (1985) recorded heart-rate and EMG. During the procedure, two of their subjects exhibited criteria of panic, in the form of a sudden rush of fear, with marked increases in heart-rate with tachycardia and simultaneous elevation of muscle tone. Clark (1988) has suggested that the relaxed state renders internal sensations more vivid. A panic response to clinically-induced relaxation arises, Clark argues, out of an attentional shift toward normal changes in autonomic activity, so that, for example, pulse-rate becomes perceived more vividly, eliciting the sudden dread of cardiac problems.

Care needs to be taken in labelling such paradoxical responses during relaxation training, since the terminology may contain misleading assumptions. Heide and Borkovec (1983) first adopted the term 'relaxation-induced-anxiety' to describe elevated anxiety levels during a deep muscle relaxation procedure. However, it is clear from the data that the subjects portraying the paradoxical effect in Heide and Borkovec's study had an anxiety attack before the procedure had been fully introduced. It is therefore unlikely that the anxiety attacks were preceded by the intended effect of the clinical procedure, i.e. relaxation, since the subjects were not relaxed at any stage of the 'relaxation' procedure. 'Relaxation-induced-anxiety' was therefore a misnomer in Heide and Borkovec's nonetheless valuable report. The anxiety attacks may have been in response to *anticipation* of the procedure's effects, in which case, the phenomenon would be more aptly named 'anxiety induced by anticipation-of-relaxation', or words to that effect.

Enigmatic data from ambulatory measures in the natural setting

Much stress has been put on panic subjects' psychophysiological crises by the authors of DSM III. Many clinical case reports cite examples of patients exacerbating levels of distress by inducing sympathetic nervous activity, often by voluntary activity, such as over-breathing and deliberate bracing of striate musculature. It is unclear, however, at exactly which point raised physiological activity actually occurs. Physiological studies using round-the-clock monitoring devices attached to the body reveal that maximum sympathetic arousal rarely coincides with the time at which subjective panic is at its peak. Panic subjects show raised baseline arousal before the onset of a panic. Nonetheless, the idea that the addition of further autonomic arousal to this already raised baseline elevates the physiological level to an intolerable peak, leading to panic, does not match the physiological data. Empirical studies often show that by the time physiology is peaking, the subject is reporting some diminution of panic levels and is beginning to calm down. Taylor *et al.* (1983) monitored eight panic subjects, only three of whom showed significantly raised heart-rate during discrete panic bouts. Moreover, Taylor *et al.* (1986) found that out of the panic attacks identified by physiological peaks, only 29 per cent were verified by the subjects.

Nocturnal panic attacks

Night-time attacks have been found to occur in around 25 per cent of panic disorder patients. The phenomenon has been described in detail by Barlow and Craske (1988), who found that over half the subjects interviewed (ten out of eighteen) reported night-time attacks to be more severe than those in the day. Both Barlow and Craske (1988) and Taylor *et al.* (1986) found nocturnal panics tended to occur in the first half of the night, when slow-wave sleep commonly occurs. The majority reported that the first sign of the attack was physiological rather than cognitive in nature. Nocturnal panickers were much more prone to fears of suffocation than their daytime contemporaries and were more likely to exhibit this fear in the daytime than panickers without nocturnal attacks.

It has been suggested that the source of nocturnal panic may be sleep apnoea, in which there is temporary retardation of breathing, followed by restlessness and rapid breathing, which does not pose a problem to non-panickers, who bring about homeostatic regulation without fully waking. Alternatively, since physical jerks tend to occur during this period of sleep, it has been suggested that these cause alarm in panic-prone individuals. Nocturnal panics do not fit the notion of hyper-vigilance to physiological swings, since they do not appear to be preceded by wakefulness, but are associated with slow delta-wave sleep. However, Clark (1988) suggests that sleep does not preclude subjects from attending to specific stimuli and gives the example of mothers, who commonly show selective attention to cries of their babies and will wake up. Even in sleep, it appears that there are 'priority channels'. Therefore, it is not unreasonable to assume that sleeping panic patients are more attentive to changes in such things as heart-rate and respiration than non-panickers.

Variability in the behavioural consequences of panic disorder

It appears that recurrent panic attacks have widely different behavioural consequences, in terms of avoidance behaviour, ranging from virtually no avoidance in
some subjects to severe avoidance, to the extent of the total disruption of pre-morbid
life style, in others. When there is marked behavioural disruption, this often takes
the form of agoraphobia. Though the popular layman's definition of agoraphobia
is a 'fear of wide open spaces', it is commonly acknowledged among clinicians that
crowds, public transport, bridges and enclosed spaces are more anxiety-provoking
(e.g. Marks 1969).

Many clinicians regard agoraphobia as a misnomer in that the syndrome is not
situationally specific enough to warrant describing the associated anxiety as
'stimulus bound'. For example, Snaith (1981) and Hallam (1985) consider the
distress in agoraphobics to be so poorly circumscribed that the term 'phobia' is not
applicable, since the presentation does not meet the criteria for phobic anxiety; after
all, agoraphobic patients become anxious indoors as well as away from home, and
tend to restrict themselves geographically because it feels safer to experience
distress in a familiar place than away from home or the hospital. Consequently,
Snaith (1981) prefers to label the syndrome 'non-specific insecurity reaction'.

There is often little difference between agoraphobia and panic disorder in terms
of psychopathology. Turner *et al.* (1986) found that agoraphobic patients and panic
patients did not differ in self-ratings of fearfulness of typical agoraphobic situations.
DSM III categorisation acknowledges that panic and agoraphobia are interrelated
inasmuch as it accommodates two sub-categories of panic disorder, namely, Panic
Disorder with Agoraphobia and Panic Disorder without. The presence of DSM
III-defined panic does not in itself predict the presence of agoraphobia.

Differences between these two clinical groups – i.e. panickers who stay away
and those who soldier on regardless – have been the subject of research since the
categories were generated. Klein (1980) acknowledges that some individuals have
panic attacks with no consequential avoidance, but puts forward the view that
virtually all agoraphobics have experienced panic attacks before the onset of an
agoraphobic episode. It would appear from Klein's observations that even panic-
attack subjects who are not agoraphobic are apprehensive and experience anxiety
in situations which are high on the anxiety hierarchy of agoraphobic patients. The
difference between avoiders and non-avoiders is not the presence or absence of
anxiety, but how the subject copes with it. There appear to be large individual
differences in degree of coping behaviour.

Predictable and unpredictable panic

DSM III(R) (1987) distinguishes between 'situational' and 'spontaneous' panic
attacks, reflecting the notion that some panics come out of the blue. Despite the
evidence, from Beck and others, suggesting that the degree to which any panic
attack is unexpected may, in actuality, depend on how skilled a subject is in locating

its eliciting stimulus, which is often cognitive, spontaneous attacks have become an important focus for biological psychiatrists.

Rachman *et al.* (1987) have devised a means by which the degree of expectancy of an attack can be measured. This is calculated for any given situation by obtaining a subjective rating of expected fear prior to exposure, and a subjective rating of actual fear during the exposure itself, from which the percentage unexpectedness is derived. Unexpected panics are more debilitating than anticipated panics and result in much more avoidance, which may go some way to explain why there are such marked individual differences in the degree of avoidance of panic subjects. Panic patients over-predict the occurrence of panic and disconfirmation often leads to fear reduction. The idea of heuristic feedback to patients, so that their own predictions can be matched with their actual reactions is likely to be beneficial in the clinical situation. Ways of delivering this type of feedback usually involve reality-testing by supported exposure to events the patient anticipates will bring on an attack.

INFORMATION PROCESSING DURING PANIC

The individual differences in avoidance/non-avoidance in response to panic may lie in cognitive components, rather than distal stimuli *per se*. Both Clark (1986) and Beck (1976) have argued that whether a given situation is construed as threatening depends on whether a subject makes a meaningful link between the situation and aspects of his/her symptom pattern. For example, Beck (1976) suggests that agoraphobic avoiders harbour specific fears of what might happen to them in crowds, enclosed spaces, high places, escalators, and while travelling. Beck claims to have traced a relationship between fears of specific situations and particular types of symptom, so that, for instance, fear of enclosed spaces is associated with suffocation and tightness in the chest.

Clark (1986) has developed this notion by suggesting that avoidance patterns in some panic disorder patients are not agoraphobic in nature because certain panic patients do not construe their idiopathic symptom profiles as being exacerbated by situations typically feared by agoraphobics. Clark provides the examples of symptoms of panic which, he asserts, may have no ramifications for an agoraphobic picture, such as nocturnal panics and fear of choking. He postulates that the presence of such symptoms is more likely to prompt avoidance behaviours specific to the mode characteristics engaged, so that relaxation and rest may be avoided as much as possible in the nocturnal panickers, and restaurants and certain foods (particularly dry foods) in the chokers, but neither avoidance pattern is particularly likely to be agoraphobic. Such predictions need validation and it may be that the more predictable the stimulus parameters of panic are for an individual, the less likely that person will be to avoid situations falling outside the situations construed as dangerous.

Unconscious processing

We have discussed how memory is sometimes retrieved by emotional cues, so that specific content of memory is more available in accordance with the prevailing felt emotion of the subject (see page 29). Clark (1988) makes the point that, typically, catastrophic misinterpretation occurs so rapidly in response to somatic changes that patients are not always aware of the means by which the catastrophic conclusion was reached. These rapidly-formed cognitions are termed 'automatic thoughts'. Automaticity implies that thinking has occurred in a reflex manner, without an intervening process of reasoning. Facilitation of the thought is said to have occurred by unconscious mechanisms of information retrieval.

It appears that shifts in attention can occur in response to impinging stimuli without the subject being aware of either the attention shift or the stimulus which has caused the shift. In a series of experiments, Mathews and colleagues have demonstrated the existence of an attentional bias in anxiety and panic patients. In a dichotic-listening procedure, Mathews and MacLeod (1985) simultaneously presented audible neutral stories via one ear and subliminal threatening and non-threatening words via the other. The subjects were required to respond as quickly as possible to words from the audible channel. The reaction time of anxiety patients to stimuli delivered via the audible channel was selectively impaired. Response latency occurred during the presentation of threatening words, but not neutral words on the subliminal channel. None of the patients was able to identify any of the words presented on the subliminal channel, yet responded selectively to the threatening words, which impaired performance on the audible task. Controls showed less selective impairment.

The selective nature of this apparent hesitancy in anxiety patients is widely interpreted as evidence of an over-preparedness to attend to specific, threatening stimuli. It is argued by Beck (1988) that it is reasonable to assume that this over-attentiveness applies to interoceptive data, such as respiration and heart-rate, as well as exteroceptive, verbal data. Referring to one of the above experiments, Beck states:

> Mathews and MacLeod (1985) . . . have demonstrated how the input of anxiety-related words through the 'unattended channel' can selectively intrude on the anxious patient's focus on another task. It is conceivable that in a similar way certain internal stimuli can draw away the panic patient's attention from other tasks – even prior to their consciously recognising the stimulus – and somewhat disrupt their conscious cognitive processes. This automatic processing of information and consequent redeployment of attention could play a role in the loosening of voluntary control over cognitive processes.
>
> (Beck 1988: 94)

Conscious processes

Both Beck (1988) and Chambless and Gracely (1989) have been impressed by the fixedness of the catastrophising thoughts during the attack itself. The fixation is at the expense of competing thoughts, some of which would otherwise counter catastrophic assumptions by offering alternative explanations.

Beck (1988) suggests that panic can be differentiated from anxiety on two counts, the first of which is the content of these fixed thought patterns. Beck postulates that when the content centres around worrisome themes which do not pertain to an imminent threat to the subject's survival, anxiety tends to be the predominant affective state. If, however, the thoughts relate to an immediate threat to personal survival, such as fatality due to accidents or sudden ill-health, panic is more likely to occur:

> when there is acute anxiety that is diagnosable as panic, the cognitive content centers on the fear of impending physical, mental or behavioural disaster. When the patient experiences anxiety but not panic, then the main cognitive theme centers on less immediately threatening problems, such as social relations, performance, and achievement. Similarly, if the fear is of some condition which is not immediately threatening to survival, such as gastrointestinal, musculo-skeletal, or kidney disease, panic is less likely to occur.
>
> (Beck 1988: 97)

The second factor which Beck considers gives panic a unique quality differentiating it from anxiety is the impervious nature of these thoughts, which during an attack are fixed and not amenable to correction or modification. The beholder is unable to dissuade himself of the validity of the conviction that he is about to die or go completely insane. Beck attributes this in part to a dysfunction of information processing, in that the panicking patient is unable to access information which would counter the cognitions of impending doom. All counterarguments to the prophecy of immediate personal disaster are unavailable to consciousness, so that there is a complete lack of internal dialogue to mitigate inaccurate, catastrophic assumptions about the meaning of the attack and the subject's immediate fate. Beck holds the view that there is a failure to retrieve from memory data which could potentially establish a more reasoned approach. The panicking subject is, in effect, cut off from rational beliefs, since counterevidence of calamity cannot be recalled into consciousness. Stored data which might be of considerable use in reducing acute distress by reasoned judgement is, in Beck's account, elusive and outside the person's perspective.

An example of the above is a patient of one of the present authors, who readily acknowledges outside of an attack that the sensations associated with the onset, such as trembling, cold sweats and palpitations, are very similar on each occasion. The patient has had many dozens of attacks, with symptoms of roughly equal quality and severity, which, for two or three hours, convince him of impending death by cerebral haemorrhage. The fact that he has experienced such sensations many times prior to the current attack somehow always eludes him and he is incapable of self-reassurance by the thought that he has survived many such identical attacks, which were of no medical significance. As each attack wanes, thoughts that he is able to calm down and will return to normality are met with considerable relief, but these thoughts are markedly absent during the course of the short-lived crisis itself. Previous experience of the outcome of attacks has no effect on the next attack because heuristic data of this nature is not brought into consciousness.

Beck (1988) regards the suspension of reflective, normalising thought processes as diagnostic of an attack. He forwards the view that since there are discrepancies between physiological output between individuals during an attack (as discussed above), the cognitive profile of an attack is a better reflection of its character. He states:

> We may find in panic attacks, as in delusions, that there is a disruption or loss of reality testing of the idée fixe. When the channels for appraising reality are re-opened (via administration of drugs or input of correct information) the patient is enabled to learn at the most fundamental level that his or her catastrophic thinking is incorrect. . . . My focus on the cognitive processes leads to a tentative thesis: The necessary condition for a panic attack is the disassociation of the higher-level reflective processes from the automatic cognitive processing. The essential feature of the panic attack is not the psychobiological activation, since some patients have panic attacks when pulse and respiration are normal.
>
> (Beck 1988: 101)

In an attempt to assess the cognitive deficit during an attack, Beck and Sokol-Kessler (1986) developed a series of fifteen items which they have termed the 'Cognitive Dysfunction Inventory'. The questionnaire differentiates Panic Disorder and Generalised Anxiety Disorder reasonably well, with panickers scoring significantly higher.

Ottaviani and Beck (1987) studied a series of thirty patients who fitted the DSM III criteria of panic, in order to examine the relationship between thought content and panic. They found that concomitant with panic, the prominent thoughts and images related to loss of control, fainting, heart attack, death, going mad, loss of breath and choking. Amplification of somatic sensation or dysfunctional self-experience in attention occurred in all patients, who attributed disastrous consequences to such phenomena.

In the same study, the antecedents of initial attacks were also investigated retrospectively. Beck (1988) has stressed that a factor exacerbating further attacks is the tendency for panic patients to be hypervigilant of interoceptive cues, particularly in situations resembling those in which previous panic attacks have occurred. As a result, minor changes in self-experience or shifts in physiological arousal become the focus of attention, around which expectations of imminent personal crisis become oriented. The observation is supported by Hibbert (1984a), who asked panic patients what their first signs of an impending attack were; 53 per cent of the sample mentioned physical sensations.

FACTORS WHICH PRECEDE THE ONSET OF A PANIC ATTACK

We have already considered the mental events which characterise the onset of a panic, including over-attentiveness to somatic changes, which are then interpreted as disastrous and incapacitating. A number of studies have looked at events which are not immediately related to the onset of panics, that is, events which are unrelated to the phenomenology of panic *per se*, but are possible predisposing factors. Borkovec (1985) has stressed the importance of worry, which he notes is present in the history in the run-up to an attack, usually for a period of several weeks. The content of worry, such as disagreements, concerns over achievements at work, marital disharmony and bereavement, may be unrelated to somatic sensations at that stage. It is difficult to draw conclusions regarding the transposition of such psychological events to panic itself. The presence of worry may generate high arousal, which becomes the source of alien somatic sensations, subsequently interpreted as catastrophic.

One of the current authors has encountered panic disorder in a compulsive gambler, whose symptoms were largely related to listening to horse races in which he had invested money. If his horse trailed behind from the outset, panic never ensued. Instead, symptoms were related to a close race, in which there was considerable suspense and hope (Fewtrell, unpublished). This example suggests a close relationship between panic and thrill, the common denominator of both being elevation of somatic cues of arousal; in panic patients, such cues are subject to considerable misinterpretation, such as the certainty of expectation of a negative outcome.

There is some clinical evidence that background dissatisfaction, in terms of marital disharmony, affects the course of agoraphobia. Bland and Hallam (1981) treated sixteen agoraphobic patients with brief behaviour therapy, consisting largely of *in vivo* exposure. The subjects were assessed for level of disability and for marital satisfaction, both before and after they had taken part in the two-week treatment programme. The results indicated that all the patients had made initial improvements in approach behaviours by the end of the two-week period. At a three-month follow-up, the patients who were in good marriages as a group maintained their improvement. However, the patients in the 'marital dissatisfaction' group dropped back, exhibiting the same level of incapacity at the three-month follow-up as before treatment. Unfortunately, the presence or absence of panic disorder is not recorded in this study, since the concept of panic disorder was introduced to the DSM III classification system around the same time that the research was carried out, though one of the authors recalls that many of subjects exhibited panic by DSM III criteria (Hallam, personal communication).

SOME COMMENTS ON TREATMENT APPROACHES TO PANIC DISORDER

Treatment approaches which can be used in mitigating a specific condition sometimes predate the conceptualisation of the condition itself. To a certain extent, this has occurred in the development of treatment approaches used in panic disorder, which were employed, largely by clinicians, in the treatment of 'anxiety' prior to 1980, when DSM III was first published.

Schultz and Luthe (1969) published a four-volume text outlining methods of 'Autogenic Training', an approach which aimed to nurture self-control techniques in the management of anxiety (1968, 3). The approach involved encouraging the patient to re-experience moments of acute crisis in the clinic and, with the aid of hypnosis, educate the patient to obtain mastery over the symptoms. The patient was then advised to apply the same self-control of anxiety in settings more akin to a typical anxiety-provoking situation.

Snaith (1981) has developed this aspect of Autogenic Training for the treatment of panic attacks by use of a procedure which he terms Anxiety Control Training (ACT). ACT involves carefully recording patients' descriptions of acute anxiety and using the same semantics to induce an attack under hypnosis. Once elicited, the hypnotherapist then instils confidence in the client during the induced attack, who is then encouraged to regain 'calm control'.

It is generally felt that panic attacks are resistant to treatment, unless the patient is shown a way to deal with the attacks when they begin. The introduction of coping strategies and mastery-based techniques, which the patient can employ *in situ*, are viewed as important. Often, clinicians have advised engineering panic sensations in the clinic, followed by a means of de-emphasising the significance of physiological and psychological symptoms (e.g. Beck 1988). There is no word-for-word package in such procedures, since the degree of physiological involvement in an attack, and the specific attributions which individual subjects give to each symptom, are variable and idiopathic. Therefore, the specific reassurance given to any one patient will be unique, but, nonetheless, there is considerable consensus in general terms.

The first problem for the clinician, following assessment, is how to elicit an attack in the clinic, and to what degree of severity. Elicitation of panic features can be carried out in a variety of ways, but mainly by use of imagery, exercise and hyperventilation, all of which have been found to produce physical sensations akin to an attack. The use of hyperventilation has become increasingly popular (see Clark 1988). There are two distinct aims of producing the simulation: first, to familiarise the patient with the associated sensations of panic; and second, to educate the subject into gaining control of the crisis, so that if encountered again, the panic features can be countered by self-regulation of breathing. In practice, these two aims overlap and various therapists recommend their own points of emphasis in forming a clinical strategy. But the common theme of most treatment packages is the regeneration of symptoms, thoughts, images and sensations similar to those which occur when the subject is in an acute crisis. When such phenomena are experienced in a 'safe' setting, such as the out-patient clinic, in the presence of a trusted and supportive therapist, then these features of panic can be reconsidered and reconstrued in the cool light of day.

Most clinicians would not disagree with this model, but widen it beyond manipulation of conditioned emotional responses to interoceptive cues, to include the manipulation of important intervening variables involved in catastrophisation. This is an area central to cognitive therapists, such as Beck and Emery (1985) and Clark (1986). These authors provide excellent source material for the practical application of cognitive treatments of panic.

The essence of cognitive treatment of panic is the modification of interpretations a patient makes about interoceptive and self-world experiences. Often, such experiences are deliberately elicited in the patient under controlled conditions in order to get the patient to reassess their significance. For example, a patient whose attacks are characterised by over-breathing, followed by unreality experiences and dizziness, can be instructed to hyperventilate in the clinical setting (usually for between one and two minutes). The aim would be to generate giddy and unreal experience in order to point out that such sensations are caused by hyperventilation *per se*, not by some kind of serious physical pathology. Clark (1988) advocates the training of controlled breathing in redressing the blood CO_2 level, and in doing so incorporates a physical as well as subjective coping strategy. Rapid self-regulation of thought and feeling states also serves to reassure the patient that deviations of physical and psychological systems from the baseline do not inevitably result in crisis, thus changing future expectancy when exposed to the same internal conditions. This process of increasing confidence in coping during periods of minor alien experiences is sometimes termed manipulation of 'self-efficacy' (Bandura 1977).

It is interesting to compare Beck's cognitive analysis of panic with the notion of *Dasein-analysis* described by Heidegger. In both, there is an emphasis on taking a snapshot of subjective processes during a specific and fleeting moment in time. In the assessment of panic, cognitive therapists often use what they have come to call the 'vertical arrow technique'. This is a method of interviewing which forms the basis of an important cognitive approach to the treatment of panic.

In the vertical arrow technique, the patient is invited to concentrate on the assumptions which are adopted during a panic attack and invited to elaborate these assumptions, by projecting forward in time and giving an account of the anticipated consequences of an attack. Beck regards the 'vertical arrow' technique as important in determining the hidden assumptions which have prompted such over-concern over interoceptive sensation. Many authors have noted that careful questioning, which is kept centred on minuscule time-frames of the panic itself, can often reveal assumptions of which the patient was only barely aware. Vertical-arrow techniques are therefore vital to self-regulation and self-counterargument, since fallacious assumptions cannot be corrected by the individual unless they are brought into full consciousness. Exposure of hidden thought premises (e.g. expectations of doom) lays bare the catastrophised rationale in consciousness, exposing it to self-reflective evaluation.

SUMMARY

The concept of panic disorder is a relative newcomer to the diagnostic system. It is marked by the theme of catastrophisation as the main feature of propositional self-statements. Panic is often regarded as a hypersensitivity to benign interoceptive stimuli, the significance of which become inflated out of proportion by the patient, who evaluates the consequences of such stimuli as powerfully noxious and life-threatening. Many cognitive therapists find that successful treatment cannot be brought about without eliciting a mini-attack in the clinic, not least because by doing so, the catastrophic propositions are accessed and therefore 'laid bare'. The essence of cognitive therapy for panic attacks is the challenging of propositions of doom and calamity in the face of minor somatic sensation, and to give the patient a sense of mastery over bodily cues.

In the following two chapters, we have chosen to concentrate on two symptoms of panic disorder which are rarely mentioned in detail, but which are important inasmuch as they illustrate some of the 'ego-dysfunction' characteristics of panic, namely, psychogenic dizziness and depersonalisation syndrome. These features reflect a distortion of self-awareness and self-world relations, and can occur singularly, or as part of a wider clinical picture. Distortions in the amplitude or authenticity of experience are factors which contribute to the dysfunctional assessment of self in relation to body and world.

Chapter 5

Psychogenic dizziness and other self-world disturbances

SOME CHARACTERISTICS OF DIZZINESS

Dizziness is a subjective experience of a change in self-world relations which is difficult to verbalise. The experience can have both physical and psychological provocations and is a feature of a wide range of organic and non-organic complaints, including anxiety. It can be experienced either as an aversive or a pleasant experience, and is an experience familiar to most people at one time or other during their lives, for example, at fun fairs.

Dizziness is frequently tied to the medical condition of vertigo and attributed to vestibular dysfunction (e.g. Brandt and Daroff 1980), but it is important to distinguish vertigo from dizziness. Vertigo results from a conflict between the different systems responsible for maintaining the constancy and uprightness of body posture. There are basically two systems compensating to keep the body constant in space: one relying on optokinetic-retinal feedback; the other vestibular, relying on the body's frame of reference. Conflicting input into these systems arises through a conflict between visual, gravitational and somatosensory cues. This conflict can be provoked by a fast movement, a lack of available cues, a sudden change in posture, a loud sound (the so-called 'Tullio phenomenon'), anticipatory anxiety or peripheral or central damage to the balance organs (Dix and Hood 1984). In most cases, the balance system can compensate for conflict, even in the case of peripheral damage, and patients can habituate to the vertigo (Drachman and Hart 1972).

The original definition of vertigo by Cawthorne (1945) was the hallucination of rotatory sensation. Nowadays, the term envelops a variety of different experiences; for example, the world may appear to spin in relation to the person, or the person may feel their head going round as the environment stands still. There are also marked differences in the speed of spinning and its duration. Sometimes, there are no complaints of spinning at all. Subjective reports of dizziness may not always include hallucination of movement, sometimes being accompanied by other somatic symptoms, such as headache, nausea, and a range of autonomic and cholinergic effects (O'Connor 1986; Beyts 1987).

Dizziness is not a coherent construct in medical terms, nor is it a unitary experience in its lay usage. Patients who describe themselves as sufferers of dizziness usually have problems specifying exactly what sensations they experience and may report a range of sensations, such as light-headedness, muzziness, feeling distant, feeling not quite themselves, vague sensori-motor symptoms and oscillopsia (objects appearing to jump from place to place). Dizziness is not associated with any set medical complaint or somatic site, which makes it difficult to classify even as a psychosomatic disorder. Brandt and Daroff (1980) list several disorders associated with dizziness, including epilepsy, ototoxicity, eye problems, vascular disease, tumour and labyrinthine dysfunction. Although the assumption in each case is that dizziness has a definite medical association, overall, the experience of dizziness has no single medical causation.

The type and incidence of the dizzy experience has not been as extensively investigated in the normal as in the clinical population. Everyone has at some time or other felt dizzy, but does not necessarily find the experience aversive. It would thus be true to speak of normal and abnormal experiences of dizziness, though the range within each category seems quite wide. Abnormal experiences of dizziness have been most closely tied to vestibular-system dysfunction. The vestibular system is, of course, the centre for co-ordinating input and output from a variety of sensory systems, including hearing, touch and muscle co-ordination. It can in a general sense be said to be responsible for maintaining the person's upright position in relation to a changing world.

Irrespective of the apparent relationship between vestibular problems and dizziness, there is little correlation between the intensity of reported dizziness and organic severity (Stephens et al. 1991), nor is there necessarily a relationship between dizziness and loss of balance or other physical consequences of vestibular disturbance (Afzelius et al. 1980; O'Connor 1986). A common factor is that all patients reporting dizziness as a problem find the sensations they experience aversive, and often the dizzy sensation can be indistinguishable from feelings of anxiety. But, interestingly, the primary preoccupations of those anxious about their dizziness are to do with fear of social embarrassment, fear of being unable to cope in public, and fear that the dizziness signals the onset of a serious medical illness. In other words, the aversiveness is more to do with the meaning or implication of the attack than with the sensations per se (Hallam and Stephens 1985; Beyts 1987).

It is widely recognised by clinicians that a substantial proportion of patients (29 per cent–40 per cent) presenting with dizziness have no organic signs (Manding 1982). Dizziness ranks seventh among particular symptoms of patients with anxiety. Seventy-eight per cent of these patients complain of dizziness. Manding reports a study of fifty patients admitted to a university hospital's 'vertigo clinic' of whom 40 per cent were neurotic, mostly with anxiety problems. Such cases are regarded as 'psychogenic' forms of dizziness, which are anxiety-related, either as concomitants of anxiety or as a substitute for anxiety sensations in stressful situations (Schilder 1933; Magnussen et al. 1977). One possible functional link with anxiety is hyperventilation, and there is an established association between dizziness and raised blood-oxygen levels (Drachman and Hart 1972). Other links with anxiety include personality effects.

Patients suffering from dizziness and balance disorders often show a characteristic personality profile which is high on neuroticism, hypochondriasis and obsessional traits (Stephens 1975). These patients are often prone to develop phobias. Freud (1957) considered that dizziness was an expression of psychic helplessness and a defensive reaction to ward off anxiety. But anxiety and dizziness also occur together and anxiety can produce vestibular disturbance, not least by producing behavioural provocations, for example, rocking or twisting, or head and neck tension, often associated with nervousness.

Despite the association between dizziness and anxiety, it is difficult to ascertain a cause and effect relationship. For example, on the one hand, Hinchcliffe (1967) suggests that Ménière's disease is precipitated by excess emotionality, while, on the other, Pratt and Mackenzie (1958) assume that vestibular dysfunction is the primary aetiological process, anxiety being secondary. There is no doubt that dizziness is in itself distressing, and as Jakes (1988) points out, not all anxiety-prone subjects are also prone to dizziness. Furthermore, Crary and Wexler (1972) attempted to identify the emotional precursors of dizziness, but failed to locate any specific antecedent life event.

Presumably, a greater emphasis on sequential analysis would be desirable to determine which sensations are antecedents and which are consequential; so far, it is not clearly established which people experience anxiety only as a consequence of their dizziness and which people experience dizziness as a result of their anxiety. Patients actually report difficulty in distinguishing the anticipation from the reality of an attack; the anticipation alone producing dizzy symptoms.

One pertinent line of enquiry is whether non-organic dizzy patients present a qualitatively different anxiety picture than those with organic problems. O'Connor et al. (1988) have observed that subjects with known peripheral vestibular lesions show a different quality of experience preceding an attack than their non-organic counterparts: the latter report significantly greater anticipatory anxiety, in terms of autonomic sensation. Non-organic subjects cannot discriminate clearly between anticipatory anxiety of an attack and the dizziness attack itself; one merges into the other. Organic subjects show a more sudden onset, with shorter and less pronounced anticipatory features. There was also a distinction reported in type of sensations experienced prior to an attack; those with damage to balance and organs tended to have more accurate and empirically-verifiable fears of falling over rather than, as in the non-organic case, just general fears of losing control.

In this study O'Connor et al. (1988) identified both the somatopsychic and psychosomatic nature of the dizziness provocation. In the psychic case, anticipatory anxiety produces either excitation or inhibition and attendant strategies of either tensing or over-breathing and hyperactivity, either of which may produce dizziness. In the somatic case some damage or disturbance produces vestibular instability, which produces secondary symptoms of anxiety.

Jacob (1988) has raised the possibility that a subgroup of panic-disordered patients may have vestibular dysfunction, the systems of vestibular dysfunction thereby triggering or reducing the threshold to panic attacks resulting in the development of panic disorders. Jacob cites a study of 17 patients in a dizziness clinic who were diagnosed as having 'psychogenic dizziness' because their vestibular test results were normal; 76 per cent had vestibular problems. In a related study, Jacob and co-workers (Clark *et al*. 1992) found symptoms related to panic in 21 out of 103 patients, with a history of panic attacks in an additional 28.

The psychosomatic/somatopsychic nature of the vestibular dysfunction is also emphasised by the link between migraine and vertigo on the one hand (Kayan and Hood 1984) and between panic and migraine on the other hand (Stewart *et al*. 1989). In view of this bi-directionality, it is difficult to sustain the hypothesis that panic and anxiety are secondary to vestibular dysfunction. Migraine can be produced by central disturbance but the most common factors are psychological ones: stress, relief from stress, anxiety, depression and emotional disturbances (Kayan 1984).

DIZZINESS AND AROUSAL

The link between dizziness and excessive emotionality is obscured by the observation that dizzy episodes sometimes occur during periods of relaxation and inactivity and fatigue (Schilder 1933; Brandt 1984; Manding 1982; O'Connor 1986). This well-established finding is consistent with the observation that dizziness can be precipitated by a switch from high to low task demand (Hallam 1985). For example, Hallam cites light-headedness occurring in an aircraft pilot after take-off, at the point when control of the aircraft was relinquished to automatic pilot.

Two case examples may serve as further illustrations. The first involved a patient who worked as a computer operator and who would suffer a short bout of dizziness when moving from her work to a more relaxing task. In the second, a teacher suffered attacks of dizziness not when teaching in a very stressful school environment, but at the weekend and on holidays when relaxing.

This high to low switch might be defined more precisely by saying that situations which provoke dizziness in these cases tend to be those in which the person is not as involved, or 'disengages' through lack of task demand. Although this link between dizziness and lowered arousal appears to contradict evidence of the link between dizziness and raised arousal, there may be a common element in both sets of findings. The two groups may both be responding to abrupt arousal shifts, whether in an upward or a downward direction.

There is a substantial change in the arousal gradient. That is to say, it is the magnitude of the change, regardless of direction, and therefore independent of whether there is an elevation or diminution in absolute terms. This would explain why both sensory deprivation and excessive stimulation exacerbate depersonalisation, and similarly, why both reduction in task demand and emotional distress precipitate dizziness.

COGNITIVE EVALUATION PROCESSES

Sudden arousal shift may produce a temporary discrepancy between cognitive processes and autonomic activity. It may be that during brief periods when internal sensation needs to be reinterpreted, and the cognitive flow is temporarily suspended in the light of sudden autonomic shift, the covert self-evaluative system is at its most vulnerable. Jakes and Beyts (1985) have found that certain cognitions can induce a dizziness attack. They report a case in which a change in the patient's beliefs about dizziness made further physical treatments unnecessary. Most of the cognitions this person had related to fearful expectations about the reactions of others to her, and her own ability to perform. Baloh *et al.* (1984) demonstrate that self-instruction and covert imagery can go some way to alleviate dizziness and associated nystagmus. O'Connor *et al.* (1989) report the case of a woman whose evaluation of her surroundings, or of the features in her surroundings, as odd and out of place provoked dizziness. Hinoki (1985) has reported that the memory of vertigo can itself cause dysfunction in equilibrium centres, since such memories may excite the adrenergic system, upsetting brain-stem co-ordinating functions.

DIZZINESS AND DEPERSONALISATION

Dizziness and depersonalization are frequently reported together, though the order of their occurrence may be unclear. The linguistic aspect of the patient's report may deserve special clinical attention. There does not appear to be a vocabulary within everyday English language to describe depersonalisation and associated phenomena such as '*jamais vu*' and autoscopy. The disturbance of self-world relations is poorly provided for in everyday vocabulary, and one of the few words in common use which refers to this general experiential area is the adjective 'dizzy'. On the basis of this linguistic deficit, it seems plausible to assume that depersonalisation symptoms sometimes masquerade as 'dizziness' complaints.

Skelton-Roberts (1975) studied 35 cases of depersonalisation and observed what he termed 'dizziness-like symptoms' in 15 of them (43 per cent). Complaints ranged from anticipation of dizziness, 'I was frightened to turn around quickly in case I was going to be dizzy'; 'I didn't like to move my head. It seemed as if the whole scene would go woosh', to direct comparisons with, or analogues of, dizziness itself, 'I'm sure there's something wrong in my head, as if there's a mass of bees in it'; 'It's like a merry-go-round at the back of my mind' (Skelton-Roberts 1975: 336). For many reasons, depersonalisation and dizziness portray overlapping properties. It is therefore not unreasonable to assume that one of these states may be mistaken for the other. There is a similarity between the two states. Depersonalisation is often experienced in cases of vestibular disturbance, for example, in 'break-off' experiences, where aviators fly at high altitudes and there is a clash of gravitational and optokinetic cues.

The similarities between dizziness and depersonalisation are that they are equally responsive to arousal gradients. They may have similar precipitating factors, and a possible vestibular link. Depersonalisation is reported in about 40 per cent of panic and agoraphobia cases. The symptoms of space phobia associated with dizziness in the elderly can include depersonalisation. The strategies used to control both are similar and involve attentional engagement, narrowing of cues, going into darkness and standing still (Charbonneau and O'Connor 1993). However, the secondary worries of each problem are distinct, with dizzy patients tending to worry that they will be a victim of their attack, or that they have a brain tumour, or will vomit and fall over. Depersonalised patients tend to worry that they are going mad, will sink into nothing, lose touch with reality, or have an accident.

There are, on the other hand, also important differences between the two states. On a pragmatic level, to the general practitioner, a complaint of 'dizziness' acts as a cue for referral to ENT, while complaints of unreality are a cue for referral to the psychiatric services, if either goes any further than the primary-care setting. In the patient, the conceptualisation of a complaint as dizziness tends to excite worries about organic pathology (for example, a tumour), whereas depersonalisation generates fears of impending loss of faculties, or fears of going mad. Both have in common the dread of loss of consciousness. Depersonalisation is a frequent accompaniment to schizoid states, whereas dizziness is seldom reported in schizophrenia (Manding 1982).

In terms of reported duration, dizziness can last a few weeks at most in unremitting form, while depersonalisation can occur constantly for several months without relief. Dizziness spells are often accompanied or followed by a sickly feeling and of imminent vomiting, actual vomiting occurring occasionally, but this is rare in depersonalisation. Ruminations concerning losing touch with reality are rare in severe dizziness but common in severe depersonalisation. Depersonalisation involves a diminution of sensation, while dizziness includes an increase in (albeit peculiar) sensation. Epidemiologically, there are no sex differences in dizziness, while there is a slight female bias in depersonalisation. The latter, but not the former as far as we know, is associated with temporal lobe epilepsy. These differences should not mask the similarities, particularly when it is borne in mind that we have been contrasting depersonalisation with dizziness *per se*, whether it be organic or psychogenic. It is likely that depersonalisation would resemble psychogenic dizziness far more than its organic counterpart, and it is this particular relationship which is of interest.

THE ROLE OF PERCEPTUAL PROCESSING

We have indicated the similarities between dizziness and depersonalisation in terms of their relation with arousal and the associated cognitive evaluations. There are also similarities in perceptual experience and perceptual styles. Dizziness results from a conflict perceived between any one of visual, vestibular, proprioceptive or cognitive sources regarding the person's sense of self in relation to the world. It is a borderline phenomenon occurring between subject and object, where the person may report the sensation occurring internally or externally. Either way, it represents a break in their relation with the world and the person often feels at the mercy of the environment.

Hallam (1985) views depersonalisation as the product of a threatened sense of self-concept, which is assailed by information it cannot accommodate. Conflicting cognitive information throws the beholder out of his familiar relation to the world, leading to a changed sense of self.

The unreality experiences associated with depersonalisation often give rise to fears of loss of identity, or the anticipation of impending loss of consciousness. Sometimes, there is a sensation of floating, which is disturbing to the subject. Bellack and Small (1978) observe that fears of loss of control can lead to a secondary anxiety attack. They illustrate a case in which feelings of loss of control resulted in secondary agoraphobia, which is consistent with the observation that depersonalisation sometimes results in a desire to cling to familiar surroundings, effectively restricting one's geographical mobility.

The phobias that are acquired by the dizziness-prone often involve avoidance of stimulus situations with ambivalent spatial-distance cues, and for this reason are collectively termed 'space phobia' (Marks 1981; Manding 1982), or 'height phobia' (Brandt 1984). According to Marks (1981), the main feature of space phobia is the need to be closed in while walking, coupled with a fear of the space around. Frequently, it is visual support that the person seeks, not actual physical support, and some patients can abolish their unsteadiness by closing their eyes. Marks differentiates space phobia from agoraphobia on the grounds that both the fear of falling and fear of open spaces without visual support is usually mild or absent in agoraphobia, whereas they are central in 'space phobia'. Additionally, space phobics seem on the whole not to be neurotic and to be more resistant than agoraphobics to exposure as a treatment. Height phobics also tend to be extremely sensitive to shifts in spatial cues and less certain in their judgement of height–distance ratios (McNab et al. 1978). This perceptual sensitivity is to the relationship between spatial cues rather than their absolute position. Important in this respect is Witkin and co-workers' development of the concept of field dependence-independence as a perceptual style and its relationship to neuro-otology.

Witkin developed his rod and frame test from an earlier body-adjustment test which showed stable differences in the subjects' ability to adjust themselves to upright in the presence of a tilted room (Witkin 1949). In the rod and frame test (RFT) the person perceptually adjusts a rod to true vertical in the presence of a distracting frame. This ability involves a sensory component (error from true vertical) and a cognitive element (dependency on frame tilt). This latter element involves an ability to overcome embedded contexts in perceptual functioning, and is a trait or style which Witkin and co-workers call perceptual differentiation. According to Witkin, 'differentiation carries implications about relations with the environment; a more differentiated system is characterised by separation of what is identified as belonging to the self from what is identified as external to the self' (Witkin and Berry 1975: 5). Vestibular problems are likely to increase error from true vertical on the RFT (Trites 1969; Ottenbacher et al. 1984).

O'Connor et al. (1989) hypothesised that non-organic dizzy people would be more frame-dependent than both vestibular and normal groups; in fact, they found them to be more frame-independent. This means they had a more differentiated sense of self in contrast to anxious patients, who tend towards field dependence (Witkin and Goodenough 1977). The implication could be that psychogenic dizziness sufferers portray a fixed, inflexible mode of perception. It is interesting to note that there is a tendency for depersonalisation-prone subjects also to portray rigid evaluative systems, though this has been observed in a social rather than visuo-spatial context, culminating in the anankastic personality. It is not known whether the rigidity of spatial perception in the dizziness-prone is a manifestation of anankastic traits, but such a relationship seems feasible: sensitivity to spatial-perceptual conflict generalises to social space, an entirely cognitive area, where issues of heightened social awareness and interpersonal conformity are important (Witkin and Goodenough 1977).

Witkin's field-dependence construct has been related to functioning in a number of areas, including memory, warning and concept attainment, but the strongest link is with social perception. Field-independent people are less confident in dealing with social and interpersonal cues, and worse at repressing threatening material (Goodenough 1976; Witkin and Goodenough 1977). So, some cognitive aspects of the sense of self-world relations relate to the experience of dizziness, and in this capacity dizziness and depersonalisation also show similarities.

This focus on perceptual style in dizziness assumes more importance when we consider that perceptual information trumps information from other sensory systems when it comes to resolving sensory conflict, and that the dizzy-prone show an over-reliance on perceptual cues to the exclusion of other cues. 'Positional' vertigo and anxiety patients also show a reliance on visual information for postural control, and as a consequence have a heightened sensitivity for visual-vestibular conflict (Black and Nashner 1984).

Yardley (1990) also noted that people with motion-sickness vulnerability were unable to screen out misleading visual information, as measured by the magnitude rod tilt against a rotating background frame. Motion-sickness susceptibility was associated with a tendency to utilise the visual system to determine orientation, even when that vision supplied misleading information. Yardley suggests that her results imply a deficiency in otolithic or somatosensory systems or in the capacity to use the information from these systems appropriately, coupled with an incomplete development of the finer aspects of sensori-motor co-ordination.

A related development in rehabilitative research is the effect that cognition, in particular, visual imagery, can have both in provoking and suppressing dizziness and vestibular, occular and spinal reflexes. Conversely, of course, anxiety can impede vestibular desensitisation, which is the chief rehabilitative strategy for patients with vertigo (Beyts 1987).

A key study was carried out by Baloh et al. (1984). The vestibulo-ocular reflex (VOR) stabilises retinal images during head movements. When a normal human subject is rotated sinusoidally in the dark the eye beats back and forth with a frequency proportional to the rotation. Barr and associates (1976) had previously demonstrated that the gain of the VOR could be voluntarily modified by humans. It could be increased if they imagined a stationary surround, and decreased if they imagined a fixed target moving with them. These authors assumed that this substitute signal could be fed into the same visual-vestibular interaction pathways used by true visual signals. Baloh *et al.* (1984) found that subjects had difficulty imagining a moving surround, but could decrease VOR by imagining a fixed light. They found, however, that the task demanded concentrated effort and concluded that imaginal localisation relies on engaging higher cortical function, not just peripheral fixation.

The involvement of high-level perceptual organisation in resolving spatial conflict is supported by Friederici and Levelt's (1987) work. These authors carried out a series of studies to determine how the cognitive representation of space helps to organise conflicting sensory cues. They found in two subjects that during weightlessness different reference systems for spatial alignment are used than under normal conditions. In weightlessness, the usual positional and gravitational cues are absent and subjects use predominantly the retinal vertical as a reference, while on earth, when standing upright, they use gravitationally-defined and body-defined vertical. These findings suggest that abstract mental representations can be imposed to guide orientation even when gravity cues are absent. Friederici and Levelt conclude that, as a precondition for fast adaptation, such interval representations have to be highly abstract and be independent of external modality-specific input. They speculate that there is a cognitive weighting of different perceptual cues and this avoids the possibility of conflicts, but this resolution process is entirely cognitive.

Cappon and Banks (1969b) have proposed a radical theory of orientational perception, according to which orientation organises sensory experience into percepts of the physical self and surrounding objects. They argue that pre-perceptual ordering of objects in the world in relation to self, in terms of time and space, is essential for adequate orientation in space. Because these orientational percepts are higher-order constructs, they are not dependent on any one sense data, and so are linked with symbolic and emotional systems. As a consequence, malfunctioning of orientational perception may co-vary with psychological disturbance. Because disorientation is linked with self-reference, they suggested that increased disorientation will be accompanied by depersonalisation. There is some evidence for this effect in some individuals, but as a general claim this link is inconclusive (Cappon and Banks 1969a).

Another approach to unravelling the higher-order control of vestibular integration is the ecological approach. Stoffregen and Riccio (1988) adopt Gibson's 'direct realism' and suggest that balance orientation is maintained through the pick-up of higher-order invariants in the environment. They make the valuable point that conventional theories of vestibular input make the assumption that the organism is static; whereas, of course, the person is constantly interacting in the environment. Organisms are, hence, always in a constant state of intersensory conflict and this requires continuous resolution.

Classical theories assume that there is a continual comparison of the body axes to some external referent. Stoffregen and Riccio (1988) suggest instead that a dynamic equilibrium with respect to forces acting on the organism is maintained by a controlled interaction between the organism and surface of support, leading to attainment of a particular kinematic state. Both force and some surface, or substance, to resist the force are necessary. But it is the action of the organism which defines the gravito-inertial force vector. Patterns of motion specify an organism's position, and the motion itself generates information flow to the visual and vestibular systems. The way information is picked up from the surface of support is crucial for the attainment of dynamic equilibrium. This information is not only higher-order invariant, i.e. to do with the relationship between muscle position and surface evenness, but is also likely to be intermodal and cut across multiple perceptual systems (touch, sight, sound, etc.). The existence of intermodal invariants increases specificity in perception and control. These authors emphasise that reliance on one modality alone is likely to increase ambiguity and conflict, which is contrary to conventional wisdom. They emphasise that information available in intermodal invariants is an emergent property (or a gestalt) in the same way that 'triangularity' is a characteristic emerging from three lines arranged against each other. They are, however, not very clear about the specific nature of the invariants that are picked up, nor how one accounts for the individual differences in pick-up. Although they emphasise the abstract intermodal nature of higher-order perceptual invariants, they do not detail whether the invariants also contain emotional or self-referenced information. But their approach follows that of Noble's (1986) ecological approach to the world of 'hearing and seeing'.

According to Noble (1986), the everyday contextual aspect of sound does not find its acoustic equivalence in laboratory settings. The audible world, as 'lived-in', contains intimate self-produced sounds, for example, the smoothish low-level intermittent rub of my pen on the page punctuated by the swishing noise of my sleeve across the paper. A variety of sounds both near and distant are always present and are to be jointly identified as personally meaningful. But it is through attention to dynamic properties and distinctive temporal patterns that we make sense of the world, and these dynamic patterns are linked to my action. As I get up, for example, the transformations in the optical structure available to my visual system occur in a predictable way and these give me perceptual feedback about myself. The optical, audible and tangible properties of the environment become transformed in characteristic ways that correlate with movements and actions.

Noble, however, introduces self and emotion as a part of perceptual relations. According to Noble (1986), the emotional tone of an utterance is crucial to its comprehension. The way a signal is presented to me is as crucial to my acceptance of it as are its contents. In addition, visual and auditory feedback from the world emphasises our self-identities. Noble proposes that the audible and visual world of communication affords maintenance of the self as an ongoing agent; I perceive myself as part of a broad environment by virtue of visual and audible horizons. But these two worlds are phenomenologically distinct. Sound is different from sight because sound must first be localised. Sight gives a finer and ever constant feedback on self-identity. Interestingly, Noble's thinking tallies with Johnson's (1988) findings in the latter's phenomenological study of perceptual processing among people afraid of the dark. Johnson noted that people prone to be afraid of the dark tended to rely almost exclusively on visual cues to establish the familiarity of an environment. But when perception is ambivalent, or not available, the imagination takes over. In this instance, relying on hearing is not of much use since hearing is time-bound and fleeting and so heightens anxiety and ambiguity.

DIZZINESS AS AN 'ACT'

The phenomenological viewpoint would also adopt an ecological position and view the experience of dizziness as a product of a perception-action coupling; that my projects in the world determine my experience. But, for the phenomenologist, there is a closer link between imagination and perception than there is in other theories. In phenomenological theory perceived reality, including spatial relations, is decided on the basis of a wider self-consciousness, including what is possible as well as what is certain. Imagination and perception are a continuum and imagination is actively involved in perception. It is against this subjective background that visuo-spatial reality appears real, and this subjective reality implies a necessary subjectivity of space. Both space and time are products of a pre-perceptual consciousness. The constancy of forms and sizes in perception is therefore not an intellectual but an existential function.

The subjectivity of space is what confronts the dizzy person most of all. The space around them contracts, or recedes into the distance, or seems to press in around them. This spatial distortion is, technically, more a change in the relations between cues, as defined by relative shifts in the perceived dimensions of open–closed space, nearness–farness of objects, and height–distance ratio (MacNab *et al.* 1978). The subjectivity of time is well recognised in the psychological literature; the subjectivity of space is not. It is well documented that when we are busy time passes quickly, but when we are bored it flows slowly. One interval may appear longer than another identical interval because more happens in the first interval. Time however is recognised as a by-product of other events. Space, on the other hand, is perceived to be a key reference point of reality and orientation. Hence, recognition of its subjectivity is more subversive. But space is subjective and, depending on my position and my focus, a room can take on a different shape. Space varies also with my state; if I am tired or excited the space may shrink. Space also depends on context; if I have a lot of people in a room the space may seem to expand and its configuration may change.

We have already noted that there seems good reason to suppose that perceptual organisation operates at an abstract level and orchestrates symbolic social and self-perception as part of spatial perception. So, it should not be surprising that a girl who suddenly feels socially out of place at a disco, because the people around feel strange, should also experience a subjective impression that the space around her is receding. A lady who feels the shoes worn by her accompanying escort are out of place with the suit he is wearing and with the taste of the rest of the social gathering feels the space between her and others shimmering and contorting.

However, in order to be coherent ecologically, the subjective change in perception of space must be tied to a change in the person's activity, as we have noted. In perception-action coupling, a subjective change in perception is coupled with a change in activity. But the kind of change in activity accompanying dizziness is far from evident. The person may be perfectly still and experience dizziness; he or she may be standing up or sitting down and doing nothing at all and be dizzy; or be performing on the same occupation before, during and after feeling dizzy. A possible solution to this enigma is that the person imagines self-action and imposes this imaginary action on their actual frame of action.

The height phobic on the edge of a cliff does not 'receive' conflicting sensory information causing them to perceive conflicting cues. The person rather acts out the possibility that he or she is actually already falling over the cliff and on the way down (to the sea). The person imagines this possibility; they and their body effectively live the falling over. The sky recedes and the ledges of the cliff pass by and the world turns round. This imaginary fall is as real for them as their actual static position on top of the cliff.

The dizzy conflict, then, is an action conflict, not a perceptual one. All the somatic symptoms reported, sweating, jittery legs, breathing problems, vertigo and the scene swirling before them, are sensations generated by a struggle between two incompatible acts; between the one act of staying on top of the cliff, and the other act of already falling off it. It is the clash between two possible worlds.

Similarly, the boy or girl in a disco who experiences visuo-spatial distortion imagines the action of escaping the disco. If s/he were to run away, the others would indeed become more distant as s/he walked further away. But s/he does not or cannot walk away, so instead imagines the action of walking away. This possible world of fleeing conflicts with the cues created by the actual world of staying. The dizzy person imagines an action, reacts to this image and then lives out the somatic and perceptual concomitants resulting from the conflict their imagination produces with the actual activity that is already underway. Typically, the person is actually in a static position but imagines some dramatic compelling action which conflicts with the actual stationary frame of self-reference. Dizziness, then, is essentially an act, not a sensation. So why would the person wish to imagine that their co-ordinates of reality are other than their current static ones?

We have already noted that the dizzy-prone rely unduly on perceptual cues. In the absence of other somatosensory cues, disturbance at a high level of self-consciousness could become translated entirely into subjective changes in spatial cues without further grounding in other frames of reference. Hence, one strategy to help overcome anticipatory anxiety would be to attend to other somatic-gravitational cues. In fact, any engagement of the person in a task which puts subjective perceptual cues in a narrower perspective can subdue dizziness. For example, focusing on a specific activity during height phobia can reduce the symptoms.

An 'act' model of dizziness incorporates several features reviewed earlier concerning the abstract representation of space in the mind: the link between social, symbolic and physical spatial representations, and the vulnerability of perceived spatial relations between self and world.

The greater reliance of this dizzy-prone group on visuo-spatial cues for self-reference, at the expense of other somatic and gravitational cues, may make it easier for the subjective change in space fully to absorb them than it would in the nondizzy-prone. The space before them is their reference point; if this changes so do they. But the role of imagination is crucial in vividly anticipating and creating the consequences of a possible activity and so playing on their perceptual sensitivity. As we saw earlier, imagination can provoke or prevent both nystagmatic reactions and subjective disorientation.

If the dizzy-prone are also high on obsessionality as the evidence reviewed earlier suggests, then they may have a greater tendency than normal to prejudge, anticipate and jump ahead and imagine consequences before they have arrived and so react to them before they have happened.

SOME SPECULATIVE THERAPEUTIC IMPLICATIONS

One of the main therapeutic implications of the psychological approach would be to focus the clinician's attention on the phenomenology of the person's account, rather than primarily on a diagnostic category, since it is only through conscious report that one can gather precisely what action is producing the somatic sentiments. The conscious experience of the sufferer and all they report about it is the key to understanding which possible 'acts' are in conflict. In other words, it may be that the thoughts, expectations and worries of the person reporting dizziness or depersonalisation may in some way play a part in defining the problem. Hence, they should be treated as important operants to be explored in ameliorating the dizziness experience, rather than dismissed as adjuncts to the 'real' physical problem.

Delving into conscious experience means finding out the exact form of the subjective distortion of space, and the precise nature of the tensions and autonomic sensations experienced. What exactly does the person imagine during the experience? What exactly are they doing?

It would not seem unreasonable to propose that the very unfamiliarity of the person with a 'dizzy' experience may be a cause of anxiety. The anxiety is augmented by a lack of vocabulary with which to describe and share the experience. More conventional cognitive approaches might also prove useful in the following way.

Unreality-prone patients commonly dread lapsing into some form of oblivion in which their faculties cease to function, while dizzy patients anticipate fainting and loss of consciousness. Therefore, a legitimate starting point of therapy might be to challenge such assumptions and to confront the patient with the lack of evidence to support his or her expectations of the consequences of the problematic experience; in other words, the identification and modification of faulty thought premises with a view to reducing the distress which the problematic experience generates. It could be useful to make the person aware of their subjectivity of space and the conditions where it changes, helping them integrate other self-reference coordinates besides perceptual cues into their 'sense of reality'. Using the imagination to modify the perceptual anticipations of their dizzy state would also be important.

An evaluation of a small-group approach to dizziness rehabilitation reported benefits from sharing subjective distortion experiences, and challenging expectations about the controllability and predictability of attacks (McKenna and O'Connor 1987).

Despite the marked dysphoria reported by dizzy patients in the clinical setting, disturbances of self-world relations are not inevitably unpleasant. Subjectively pleasant forms of both depersonalisation and dizziness can easily remain unacknowledged by the clinician, since the clinician's role is to attend to the casualties rather than the connoisseurs of such experiences; and yet, following on from this point, not all forms of dizziness are unpleasant. Fairgrounds are full of devices which toss and whirl their delighted passengers around and around while onlookers queue gleefully for the same disorienting experience. These subjects do not crowd the clinics in search of an antidote to the subjective sensations they have actively sought out; yet one might wonder about the difference in quality of such experiences compared with those anxiously discussed in the clinic. The difference may lie more in the evaluation of the experience, as an emotion, than in the presence or absence of the pure sensation *per se*.

SUMMARY

Complaints of dizziness are common in ENT clinics. The medical profession has tended to view dizziness as a product of vestibular dysfunction. However, dizziness is essentially a psychological experience for which there is no one-to-one equivalent in the soma. Dizziness, like depersonalisation, bears an ambivalent relationship to arousal, but does have distinct visuo-spatial associations. It is suggested that a higher order perceptual schema integrates symbolic and physical representations of self-world space, and that dizziness is actively produced by the physical reactions to a cognitive conflict between such possible schema.

Chapter 6

Dysfunctional self-awareness – depersonalisation phenomena

Self-awareness of internal psychological events, including the self-monitoring of our perception, physical actions and of the act of thinking, are crucial to adaptive existence. As well as the content of such activities, the appreciation that it is 'I' who is performing them is crucial. Otherwise there can be no appreciation, for example, of the difference between perception of imagery and of the simultaneous external events which are taking place in the world around us. The breakdown of this discrimination between awareness of self-initiated psychological activity and events which take place in the external world results in a distortion of reality in its generally-accepted sense. Mechanisms of self-awareness are therefore of considerable importance.

JASPERIAN CONCEPTS OF SELF-AWARENESS

Jaspers (1963) listed four components of self-awareness, as follows:

1 Awareness of the boundaries of the self

Normally, human beings possess the ability to draw a distinction between self and outside world. This is the ability to differentiate between what comes from within oneself and what exists externally. For example, I know that my hand reaches out to touch the table cloth. I can feel the texture of the cloth. The feeling is mine, yet the table cloth is not part of me, but external to myself; I can conjure up a scene in my imagination and I know that I have imagined the scene, which is therefore part of my subjective space. It does not exist in front of me, but is an aspect of my consciousness. This discrimination between the 'I-ness' and things outside of me breaks down in severe dysfunctional states. In the functional psychoses, a breakdown of ego boundaries which draw the line between self and world is sometimes vividly portrayed. For example, Fish (1985) quotes a schizophrenic patient who observed a carpet being beaten and asked 'Why are you beating me?' (page 86). In ecstatic states, subjects describe 'merging with the universe', and are convinced that the self is no longer contained within subjective space. The phrase may reflect a range of experiences, including those of hypomanic patients and those valued by practising Buddhists. The breakdown of self-world boundaries is also seen in the experience of thought broadcasting, during which the patient feels that his thoughts can be heard by others. When thought broadcasting occurs, the patient has no appreciation that subjective events are private, so that inner experience is psychologically transformed into an external event.

2   Awareness of identity/continuity of self over time

The content of everyday emotional and intellectual experience inevitably changes, as do the distal stimulus situations to which we are exposed. Nonetheless, the integrated individual identifies himself/herself as a singular entity, so that there is continuity of self through time. This sense of continuity is lost in some forms of drug-induced intoxication, such as LSD and mescaline, as it is in some individuals fitting the DSM III criteria for schizophrenia. The individual may feel transposed, metamorphosed into another individual or believe that he or she has changed into an inanimate object. In severe depression, there is a disturbance in the sense of continuity and the patient may get the impression of eerie stillness and a feeling that existence has stopped. Sometimes the patient may hold a delusional belief of having turned into nothing or that the body is an empty shell. Such convictions are technically described as nihilistic.

Minor disturbances of identity can occur, such as during religious conversion. However, these shifts in identity do not normally resemble a total discontinuity of identity, however profound the personal change. Existential shifts of this kind are experienced as occurring within a temporal context, of what is experienced now and what was experienced before, by me, the same person.

3   Awareness of unity of the self

This form of self-awareness reflects the subject's appreciation of the fact that, at any one time, he is one person acting in unison, with one consciousness. Disorders of the sense of unity described in the literature include multiple personality, in which more than one personality structure and value system is present at any one time. Abse (1982) suggests that where there is a splitting of identity, as in 'dual personality', the subject, as person A, is able to comment on himself as person B, often disparagingly. Often, one 'personality' is able to comment on the other, but not vice versa. This partial disassociated state is met with considerable scepticism by many psychopathologists. Some psychoanalysts consider the phenomenon to be a means by which the ego deals with massive superego problems, so that a relatively less-repressed identity is adopted, but fails to be integrated into the personality structure. One mode of being is thus divorced from the other, so that personal responsibility in terms of guilt is not experienced during periods of acting out of the more spontaneous repertoire.

Another disturbance in the unity of self is autoscopy, in which there is an hallucination of one's own body and the site of perceptual processing is experienced as outside of the physical self. Sims (1988) points out that such experiences are rare and tend to be accompanied by a loss of familiarity with oneself. A distinction can be drawn between out-of-body experiences, in which the physical self is 'seen', projected in three-dimensional space, and desomatisation, in which the subject feels strangely out of touch with the sensations and activities of the body. In the latter, there is no hallucinated physical self, but the subject feels a distinct lack of familiarity with the physical being and might wonder if there has been a severing of the links between mind and body. Some states of profound relaxation and meditative experiences may produce this sensory impression, as discussed elsewhere in the book.

4   Awareness of activity

When carrying out a particular physical action, I sense that I am moving my own body. When I see, hear or think about something, I feel intuitively that it is me who is engaged in these mental activities. When there is a disturbance of this self-monitoring process, I may feel that it is not me carrying out the action, since I may feel divorced from the operation. Faced with this apparent contradiction, some psychotic patients conclude that they are automaton, or they are two people, the doer and the initiator. Such disturbances are likely to be related to disorders of the sense of unity, in that I do not feel it is me. Jaspers (1963) includes in this category the awareness of perceiving and of thinking. Awareness of being is usually taken for granted by a normal functioning individual, but is conspicuous by its absence in severe depression. A severely depressed patient may express the belief that 'I do not exist anymore. My insides are gone and my mind is an empty shell. Nothing is left'.

Awareness of one's own activity of perception involves the feeling that it is 'I' who is hearing, seeing, touching, etc. I feel I am the participant in my own sensing of the world. Similarly, I know that I am thinking and that the thoughts are part of my mental activity. The feeling of awareness of activity corresponds with Summerhoff's concept of 'awareness of awareness'. Summerhoff (1990) draws a distinction between awareness of stimulus events, awareness of self, and what he calls a 'reflective awareness of that awareness'. The impression that it is I who is conscious may be an irreducible feeling of authenticity of experience, which in day-to-day activity is taken for granted.

In schizophrenic thought disorder, thinking is felt to be alien to the patient, so that thoughts do not seem to come from within. This subjective disturbance of the thinking process is described by Schneider (1959) as passivity of thought; the patient feels that cognitive processes are no longer under his control and that he has no ownership of them. From the patient's perspective, thinking does not feel as if it arises from his own person and, often, delusional beliefs are constructed in order to explain the occurrence of this conscious cognitive activity in which he does not feel he has played a part. However, this lack of authenticity in one's own mental and physical actions, which Dixon (1963) terms 'self-alienation', generates a series of problems, often observed in the absence of affective disorder and in subjects who otherwise function normally. It is to this category, the so-called 'depersonalisation phenomena', which we turn next.

THE DEPERSONALISATION SYNDROME

Depersonalisation is a subjective state of unreality in which there is a feeling of estrangement, either from a sense of self or from the external environment. Afflicted individuals may complain of feeling out of touch with themselves, so that both thought and actions do not feel as if they are their own. As a result, the person may describe feeling like an automaton, robot-like and detached. It is often accompanied by minor sensory distortions, particularly of the size of external objects. Familiar items can appear to take on a novel quality, as if they had never been encountered before.

Depersonalisation can easily be overlooked by the helping professions because of its covert nature and because many people have difficulty describing such feelings. Schilder (1933) describes the state experientially in the following way:

> To the depersonalised individual the world appears strange, peculiar, foreign, dreamlike. Objects appear at times strangely diminished in size, at times flat. Sounds appear to come from a distance. The tactile characteristics of objects likewise seem strangely altered, but the patients complain not only of the changes in their perceptivity but their imagery appears to be altered. Patients complain that they are capable of experiencing neither pain nor pleasure; love and hate have perished with them. They experience a fundamental change in their personality, and the climax is reached with their complaints that they have become strangers to themselves.
>
> (Schilder 1933)

The concept of depersonalisation has a moderately long history, dating back to the nineteenth century; it was first acknowledged in name by Dugas and Moutier (1911). Depersonalisation is a subjective concept which describes an unpleasant change in the quality of consciousness, in which there is a curious change in self-experience. There is a reduction of intensity of feeling, and the beholder often complains of being dazed or woolly-headed. This is accompanied by a reported inability to feel emotion, so that the individual feels strangely cut-off and distant. This out-of-touch feeling flavours perception of the outside world so that objects may appear different, sounds muffled and colours weaker. There is generally no loss of acuity or decline in sensori-motor performance, though, ironically, deper-sonalised subjects sometimes assess their state as being conspicuous to others. Some afflicted individuals worry about the feeling of being 'alone in a crowd' and that this is the beginning of an ostracisation process leading to rejection by peers.

There is often an impression of being 'shut off' as if separated from the outside world by a glass screen. Depersonalised people usually describe themselves as taking on the role of apathetic spectator, as if they were not involved in the everyday events surrounding them. Despite this, depersonalisation *per se* does not lead to a reduction in performance, nor is it akin to Seligman's (1975) notion of 'learned helplessness'. A major difference from learned helplessness is that in the depersonalised state, there are no gross measurable changes in behaviour, while Seligman's concept involves a marked reduction in the subject's interaction with the environment. Theoretically, Seligman's concept is intrinsically related to depression. Depersonalisation, on the other hand, is not. That is not to say that depression and depersonalisation are totally independent, and it would be incorrect to state that there was no relationship whatsoever between the two states. Experienced clinicians have observed both a negative and a positive relationship between affective disorder and depersonalisation. Anderson (1938) has noted that there is a marked absence of the depersonalised state in hypomania, while in clinical depression the state often appears in accentuated form (Ackner 1954; Sedman 1970).

Over the years, claims have been made to link depersonalisation experiences to other clinically meaningful entities, particularly schizophrenia (Rosenfeld 1947), temporal lobe epilepsy (Harper and Roth 1962) and phobic anxiety (Roth 1960). Apart from hypomania, the other notable exceptions, in which depersonalisation is rare, or at least rarely complained of, are gross organic brain disease (Sedman 1970) and paranoia (Sedman 1970). However, Davison (1964) stressed that it can occur as an isolated feature in the absence of any other psychopathology and the current opinion seems to be that depersonalisation is linked to many slight shifts in the quality of consciousness. Both Roberts (1960) and Dixon (1963) have observed that roughly one-third of the university student population have experienced at least brief episodes of depersonalisation at one time or another, and this is borne out by a more recent study by Trueman (1984). These latter authors leave no doubt that depersonalisation is a common feature of everyday experience, which is therefore likely to occur in a significant proportion of clients seeking counselling, regardless of the severity of the presenting problem.

Depersonalisation is an elusive phenomenon in the sense that it involves a strange absence of feeling and an apparent reduction of vividness and reality. It is therefore difficult for many people to articulate. Whereas most subjects can readily describe an anxiety bout or feelings of morbid depression, a curious state of non-being is much more difficult to put into words. Many people in counselling do not report the experience spontaneously, but will readily describe feelings of unreality when prompted, i.e. when the subject is broached by the counsellor or clinician. It is frequently observed that clients use the prefix 'as if' to describe the experience; for example, 'It was as if I wasn't there', or 'My body seemed as if it was separate from me'. The impression of detachment which underlies the depersonalised state is described by people in different ways, and this may imply various subtypes of the same basic state. Some subjects emphasise an impression of separation from the external world – for example, 'As if I was miles away even though I was aware of what was happening'. This is a typical statement expressing the experience of derealisation, in which there is a sense of detachment from the immediacy of the external environment. The subject feels somehow removed and estranged from the surrounding stimuli, which, though comprehended, seem to take place in a dreamlike atmosphere. Other subjects complain of a qualitatively different state in which there is a remoteness from a sense of self – 'I felt myself going through the motions but felt I wasn't there at all'; 'There is a me, but I feel like it's not me, like I'm not part of me at all'. This is usually termed 'depersonalisation proper', or, simply, 'depersonalisation'. Sometimes there is a sense of physical detachment from the body (desomatisation), so that, for instance, the arms and legs can feel as if they somehow do not belong; in marked desomatisation, subjects typically complain of the body feeling as if it consisted of concrete or stone, or feeling hollow and empty.

There is some confusion over the terms 'depersonalisation', 'derealisation' and 'desomatisation', but it is generally felt in phenomenological circles that the complaints which represent each specific sub-type arise from the same form of experience. Scharfetter (1980) points out that in all forms of the disorder (collectively known as 'depersonalisation phenomena'), there is a shortcoming in what Jaspers (1963) terms 'awareness of activity'. Since this subdued awareness includes an impression of diminished authenticity in what is perceived, the external world may feel as unfamiliar as one's own thoughts and feelings. Therefore, the complaints accompanying depersonalisation phenomena may consist of the world appearing remote, or the body feeling alien, or the personality inexplicably changed. The content of the complaint reflects the subject's perceptual style and attentional bias. The core experience is the diminished sense of ownership of one's own perceptual experience, whether the object of perception is internal or external.

Depersonalisation sometimes accompanies other states. When the state appears alone, in the absence of any other aberrant mood or sensation, it is known as 'primary depersonalisation'. The presentation of the state in primary form is relatively rare in the clinic, since there is usually another picture accompanying it. However, epidemiological studies strongly suggest that primary depersonalisation is commonplace among the non-clinical population (Dixon, 1963). The factors which prompt subjects to seek professional help are unclear, but one of the major differences between people who live with the experience in an undisturbed fashion and those who seek clinical intervention is probably its frequency and duration.

It should be emphasised that, in primary depersonalisation, the interpretation of the experience never takes on delusional proportions, in that there is never an accompanying belief of being actually physically separated or removed from one's soma, cognitive processes or external world. Rather, the various forms of depersonalisation represent different modes of perception in which the vividness of experience appears somehow watered down. The frequent and typical use of the prefix 'as if' implies that the subject is using analogies to describe subjective sensation, which should not be taken to mean that the subject adopts the premise in the literal sense. For example, the statement, 'It is as if I don't exist anymore', indicates that the beholder knows that, in objective terms, he or she is still very much in the world, but that, at the same time, their knowledge of existence is not confirmed by inner sensation, which is strangely lacking. The absence of delusional content holds for depersonalisation *per se*, but it is possible that when other states are superimposed on the syndrome, an interaction effect takes place which may give rise to specific cognitive aberrations which cannot be explained by the cognitions of either state alone. Superimpositional effects are discussed later in this chapter and in subsequent stages of the book, particularly Chapter 8.

There is a clear distinction between depersonalisation and out-of-body experiences, in that the latter involves perceptual experience which emanates from outside the actual physical being. This does not occur in depersonalisation, in which there is a quality of remoteness but not removal or transfer from the physical self. In the depersonalisation process, psychological events are oriented from within the real self, whereas in out-of-body experience, psychological events are felt to occur from outside the space which the physical self occupies.

Some writers have observed that a majority of depersonalised subjects are female, and that the more intelligent one is the more likely it is to occur. While it is conceivable that women tend to be more prone to such feelings than men, the present authors question the link with intelligence. Self-experience is a complex phenomenon to describe. A relatively high level of intellect may enable the client to voice such complaints, while those clients who are of lesser intelligence are less likely to introspect sufficiently to report the complaint spontaneously. The inability to articulate an introspective event does not necessarily imply the absence of the event itself. Various authors have remarked on the enthusiasm and spontaneity with which depersonalised subjects describe their experiences in detail, once the topic has been introduced. It does seem that for some subjects, reflecting on their depersonalisation experiences is extremely difficult until they are 'cued in' to the sensation, often by a passing remark or casual question from the therapist.

Arousal criteria and depersonalisation

The most illuminating experimental studies of arousal in depersonalisation have been carried out by Kelly and Walter (1968) and by Lader and Wing (1966). Kelly and Walter examined eight cases of depersonalisation, taking measures of subjective anxiety, and also using the physiological criterion of forearm blood flow. During the depersonalised state, subjective anxiety was high, forearm blood flow was low, the latter measure distinguishing the depersonalised group from a group of other anxiety-neurotic subjects. The findings suggest that, though depersonalisation is subjectively distressing, there is no accompanying increase in physical tension. This finding is supported by Lader and Wing (1966) who happened to be taking psychophysiological recordings from a young patient when, as she lay on the couch, measures of a galvanic skin response (GSR) spontaneously diminished, giving a flat recording. The young woman subsequently remarked that she was experiencing feelings of unreality resembling a depersonalised episode, and this episode coincided with reduced physiological output.

The prevalence of depersonalisation raises the question of whether it has survival value. Mayer-Gross (1935) viewed depersonalisation as an automatic reaction comparable to the characteristic motionlessness, or death-mimic response, in animals in the face of danger and physical threat. There are many anecdotal descriptions of acute depersonalisation occurring in humans during calamitous circumstances, leading, for example, to a state of indifferent detachment in war-time (Noyes and Kletti 1976). This may suggest that the state has a survival function in provoking a kind of protective disassociation in the face of trauma. Roth (1960) considers this a common reaction to phobic anxiety.

The advantages of such disassociation are illustrated by Mayer-Gross *et al.* (1969), who cite the example of a psychiatrist who was involved in a traffic accident on his way to work, during which he exhibited a spontaneous shift in the direction of the depersonalised mode.

> The man in question was driving home at some speed on a wet road surface and as he cornered fast the car skidded. He immediately experienced a dream-like detachment and found himself steering mechanically and aware of his actions as if he were contemplating some unfortunate victim from a distance. After spinning round several times and narrowly avoiding oncoming traffic, the car finally came to a halt facing in the opposite direction. The driver felt quite calm but when bystanders spoke to him their voices seemed muffled and the surrounding countryside appeared still, remote and unreal. His own voice sounded unfamiliar. He drove on feeling quite calm, arrived at his clinic and rang for his first patient. As the patient entered the psychiatrist's depersonalisation suddenly lifted and he became aware that he was perspiring and trembling severely and his heart was pounding at a rapid rate.
>
> (Mayer-Gross *et al.* 1969)

The occurrence of perspiration and trembling in the above case can be interpreted in two ways: either the subject had exhibited such autonomic responses from the outset of the traumatic event and was unaware of them, or the sympathetic autonomic activity had not occurred until the unfortunate psychiatrist perceived himself to be out of danger and away from real threat.

There is remarkably little evidence from physiological studies to illuminate the arousal status of depersonalisation, though the data from Kelly and Walter (1968) and Lader and Wing (1966) point to inhibition of sympatheic autonomic activity, rather than lack of awareness of an elevated physiological output. The findings of Kelly and Walter and Lader and Wing would suggest that depersonalisation is linked in some way to a reduction of physiological output rather than the reduction of *awareness* of high output, since their observations point to a diminution of physiological activity during the depersonalised state. However, as in the individual case quoted by Mayer-Gross *et al.* (1969), we do not have sufficient evidence to disconfirm either hypothesis, and it raises the question of whether depersonalisation is always accompanied by a reduction of physiological arousal, or whether under some conditions there is simply a reduction in the awareness of physiological arousal, while the classic fight–flight reaction remains in operation.

Nowadays, the feasibility of depersonalisation being an adaptive rather than maladaptive response to social pressures is worth consideration; as society becomes more sophisticated, exposure to physical dangers which require a fight or flight reaction for survival are less prevalent than in the days of our ancestors, when wolves roamed the land and dangers from predators were rife. Threat in the present age has taken on a new meaning, in which the danger of physical injury from attack is rarer and less commonly requires a fight or flight response. This is particularly so in the Western world, where even wars depend not so much on physical strength as on technical ability and the formation of strategy. In many ways, therefore, the flight and fight reactions which we have inherited from our forebears are of less utility, and in some respects can be disadvantageous. For example, hyperventilation can be construed as a preparation for violent physical action, when the expenditure of physical effort does not follow. Manifest physical aggression or running away in the face of psychological threat can lose a person their livelihood, and the inhibition of fight and flight is by far the more common response to provocation than its enactment.

We are all aware of the unpleasant nature of unwanted physiological sensation during irritation with a colleague or nervousness before an examination. The sympathetic CNS involvement is of no value in such circumstances, and it is feasible that depersonalisation phenomena, with their arousal-reduction properties without loss of alertness and preservation of ongoing intellectual functions, may be a means of countering what now appears to be a maladaptive physiological response of no value. It is not difficult to appreciate the adaptive nature of detachment and truncated emotional response to curb overarousal, particularly when it is 'safe' to do so.

Shorvon (1946) and Sedman (1970) have observed that depersonalisation often accompanies relaxation, following intense or prolonged stimulation or stress. Many overworked teachers will be familiar with such feelings when there is a sudden break for half-term or bank holidays, as will hard-pressed students at the end of examinations: what should have been a state of relaxed bliss often turns out to be a vaguely unpleasant numbed frame of mind in which surroundings seem far away and in which the individual feels oddly removed from their immediate situation.

Shorvon (1946) published a review paper shortly after World War II which graphically illustrated the obscure relationship between depersonalisation and life-threatening danger. He cited examples of patients who had developed depersonalisation, often of lengthy duration, at the point at which exposure to stress had receded, such as in soldiers waiting for demobilisation after war. A patient who had lived through the bombing of London during World War II was temporarily evacuated to the safety of the countryside and became depersonalised following the move. Of another interesting case, Shorvon wrote the following:

One young man had been almost continuously depersonalised for eight years. He said he felt worse when relaxed and all right if occupied. He supposed he was the only person who would welcome, for instance, a fire, as the excitement would relieve his symptoms. The happiest period of his life was when the

Gestapo were after him and he was hiding or moving about, living on wheat ears or dry meat. He was symptom-free then.

(Shorvon 1946: 41).

Such ecological accounts provide fascinating examples of the juxtaposition of unreality feelings and exposure to stressor situations. It would appear that, where the depersonalised state is already present, exposure to stressful situations alleviates the state, at least in some individuals. Also, if there has been exposure to overstimulation or stress over a long period, depersonalisation occurs when the stressor is removed.

These observations suggest that depersonalisation is the obverse of anxiety, though other evidence points to a more complex interaction between the two states: though depersonalisation is predominantly a low-arousal state physiologically, subjective events are more complex. The state of unreality can lead to a fear of loss of identity or anticipation of loss of consciousness. Though unfounded, such fears can provoke a secondary anxiety attack (Bellak and Small 1978). Some authors postulate that despite the potential stress-inoculation function, subsequent distress, owing to fears of loss of control or loss of reality arising out of the ensuing impression of detachment, can be incapacitating in their own right, leading to restricted movement and a desire to cling to an environment which is familiar (Mayer-Gross et al. 1969: 121).

Bellak and Small (1978) cite a case in which depersonalisation resulted in secondary anxiety and subsequent agoraphobia. Interestingly, this is a direct reversal of the traditional view that depersonalisation is the consequence of an anxiety state (see Roth 1960): the depersonalisation in Bellak and Small's example is the cause rather than the effect of the phobic state. A similar temporal sequence is reported by Moran (1986), who described a series of six cases in which depersonalisation first occurred while using marijuana and subsequently continued without use of the drug. These patients presented with panic attacks and agoraphobia and, though Moran is careful to avoid the assumption that primary depersonalisation caused the phobic features, the sequence of psychological events supports the assumption that unreality feelings played a role in the restriction of geographical mobility in all six cases.

It is possible that one reason for the recent rekindling of interest in depersonalisation phenomena is the changes in DSM categories. DSM III (1987) distinguishes between anxiety and panic disorder; depersonalisation is one of the ten defining characteristics of panic. Beck (1988) prefers to emphasise the cognitive processes of panic rather than the physiological features. One reason for this is that some subjects who fit the DSM III panic criteria show little or no aberration of physiological state, even during the peak of an attack. As discussed in Chapter 4, Beck prefers to define panic disorder in terms of cognitive style. He is impressed by the conviction with which patients believe internal somatic sensations are a signal of personal catastrophe. Often, the internal sensations on which these negative cognitions are based are linked to palpitations or sensorial changes associated with hyperventilation. However, the fact that elevation of physiological state is not always recorded during panic disorder raises the question of what prompts panic attacks in such cases. Since depersonalisation has been observed in the context of physiological flattening, the state may have a particularly significant role in those panic subjects in whom physiological shifts are absent.

Though there is little known about the specific contribution of the depersonalised state to panic-disorder cognitions, there is a considerable amount of literature devoted to the cognitions of patients with primary depersonalisation, which may shed some light on the issue. Such patients are painfully introspective, and preoccupied with the apparent reduction of sensation and vividness of perception. Fears of breakdown of the faculties are commonplace, so there is a dread of losing touch with the external world completely. Owing to the dread of cessation of the sensory receptors or the processes of awareness, the beholder may anticipate the gradual fading of the sensorium, culminating in a quiet stillness akin to sensory deprivation. Some primary depersonalisation subjects anticipate with dread a situation of becoming cut off, isolated in a world of their own, not unlike the deaf-blind Rubella subject. The depersonalised state is, by definition, unpleasant and dysphoric, particularly if prolonged. Though it is now generally accepted that primary depersonalisation is not a delusional phenomenon, ironically, many depersonalised people feel they are losing their grip on reality and going mad. Such people are best reassured as, in the authors' experience, worrying about the condition and subsequent prolonged periods of introspection only exacerbates the feelings of detachment.

Some helpful strategies

To counter catastrophic cognitions, it is useful to inform the patient that about one-third of the population experience unreality feelings from time to time. It is sometimes helpful to give examples from the literature or to quote fellow sufferers; there are many illustrative examples in clinical texts on the subject. It is perhaps because depersonalisation experiences are so difficult to describe that direct quotes from subjects are readily available in publications on depersonalisation. Since it is such a complex experience to describe, many authors have relied greatly on accounts given by their patients.

Though one of the present authors has attempted the direct manipulation of depersonalisation, for the present, it appears best to avoid attempts to change the state directly and instead to encourage an acceptance of the experience for what it is. A good phenomenological analysis carried out with the client is often a useful adjunct to counselling or psychotherapy, and it is important that the clinician or counsellor indicates some prior knowledge of the state, since this alone can alleviate a great deal of distress – depersonalisation, by its nature, is difficult to describe and, therefore, when the topic is broached, many clients who have such experiences are being given their first opportunity to articulate the subjective sensations, resulting in great relief.

The depersonalised state does not generally require relaxation as the therapeutic goal. In routine clinical work carried out over a five-year period, Fewtrell (1984) noticed that response to deep muscle relaxation in forty subjects (usually in preparation for desensitisation of phobic anxiety) varied considerably. The majority of subjects found the technique pleasant and calming; some found it benign in its effects; while Fewtrell abandoned the relaxation approach altogether with seven of the subjects, owing to reported adverse reactions. Two or three subjects felt frightened by the approach, and five of the seven complained of feeling vague or in a trance-like state. On looking retrospectively at the psychiatric case notes, the presence of depersonalisation was specifically mentioned in five out of the seven subjects, while feelings of unreality were referred to in the sixth, and 'fuzzy-headedness' was quoted in the seventh. Therefore, of these seven subjects, at least five, and probably all, had records indicating the presence of depersonalisation, most commonly in the recent past. The information was derived from psychiatric interviews conducted prior to relaxation training. Unfortunately, because the clinical exercise did not start out as a research project, the case notes of the remaining thirty-three were traceable with difficulty, and at the time it was decided to obtain the notes of a random sample of ten of the relaxation-favourable patients for comparison, none of which made any reference to features resembling depersonalisation phenomena. Patients from both groups were sent the 'Self-Alienation Questionnaire' (Dixon 1963), the only rating schedule then available to measure depersonalisation. The mean self-alienation scores for the two groups were significantly different, with the relaxation-adverse group exhibiting a higher degree of depersonalisation.

The relationship between response to relaxation training and presence of depersonalisation is consistent with the observation of Lader and Wing (1966) that depersonalisation is a state of low rather than high arousal. Further attempts at arousal reduction, from an already low arousal baseline, may perhaps detract from feelings of awareness, particularly in the absence of cognitive restructuring. Arousal-reduction methods may well exacerbate depersonalisation. It would be of considerable interest to investigate the effects of states of relaxation in depersonalisation-prone subjects. Many young chronically-depersonalised subjects, particularly males, are sensation-seekers and report the absence of symptoms when placing themselves in danger (for example, while driving recklessly). It is possible that the motive for doing so is not so much hedonistic thrill as the avoidance of feelings of detachment.

Precipitants of depersonalisation stemming from environmental or life-style factors include fatigue, alcohol intoxication and withdrawal, bereavement, benzodiazepine withdrawal, LSD intoxication, cannabis intoxication, excessive caffeine consumption, sudden trauma and injestion of phenothiazines (Sedman 1970). The emotional numbness of which many patients diagnosed as schizophrenic complain is sometimes attributed to the schizophrenic condition; it is also true that the medication itself can have a depersonalising effect. Transcendental meditation is also a known precipitant, and participants of the technique are prepared in advance for such experiences in that they are taught to accept and value them. However, both meditation and relaxation tecniques should be introduced with the greatest of care in subjects who are depersonalisation-prone.

RELATIONSHIP BETWEEN DEPERSONALISATION AND OTHER PROBLEMS

Depersonalisation and schizophrenia

There was a a particular interest in depersonalisation syndrome in the 1940s and 1950s, since it was described as a 'precursor state' from which a schizophrenic picture developed. This was largely because many authors noted that patients with an insidious onset of severe mental health problems experienced prolonged periods in which depersonalisation was prominent. Lewis (1967) commented that depersonalisation phenomena should be regarded as the initial signs of a psychotic breakdown. However, the vast majority of people who experience depersonalisation phenomena do not go on to develop symptoms of schizophrenia, even when the depersonalised episode is of lengthy duration. This observation cast considerable doubt on the role of depersonalisation as an active schizophrenogenic process. Nowadays, depersonalisation *per se* is not regarded as part of the pathogenesis of schizophrenia and is considered to be of little diagnostic significance in a nosological system of the psychoses.

Meyer (1956) has pointed out that in both depersonalisation and schizophrenia there is a fading of boundaries between self and world. In depersonalisation, self-initiated activity is often felt as mechanical, with diminished ego-involvement. For example, subjects may feel estranged from their own thinking or voluntary body movement. However, the belief that one's voluntary movement is controlled from an outside source or that one's thoughts are being implanted, though frequently seen in schizophrenia, is never observed in depersonalisation. The depersonalised patient may talk of the impression that self-induced activity does not feel self-induced, but the sense of estrangement from psychological or physical activity fails to give rise to the conviction that thinking and movement have somehow been taken over. The depersonalised patient may complain of feeling as if he or she were taking no part in voluntary activity, but the knowledge that voluntary activity is self-induced and remains under volitional control remains intact.

We have mentioned earlier that disorders of self-awareness occur in the majority of psychological problems and that disorders of the awareness of activity are evident in both depersonalisation and the first-rank symptoms of schizophrenia. In the latter, Schneider (1959) describes the concept of alienation of thought, in which thinking is felt to emanate from a source outside of the individual. The schizophrenic patient may be convinced that he is not participating in his own thinking and feels that he is the recipient of thoughts, over which he has no control. This is known as a passivity symptom, which differs from depersonalisation in that the depersonalised subject feels able to alter the flow of thought, even though there may be a feeling of lack of authenticity and emotional indifference to such cognitive processes. While in schizophrenia the patient may search for the source of these apparently alien thoughts and conclude that they are being inserted by telepathy or radar, the depersonalised subject knows that his thoughts are his own, but does not feel emotionally involved in them. For the depersonalised subject, thinking may appear mechanical and devoid of emotional meaning, but the self-alienation typically provokes painfully excessive introspection, usually concerning issues of self-identity and life's meaning. There is little or no change in the flow of thought in depersonalised subjects, with the exception that fantasy may be stunted. In contrast, patients exhibiting Schneider's (1959) first-rank symptoms may become preoccupied with the idea that their thoughts are being implanted by an outside agency.

Anxiety

The relationship between depersonalisation and anxiety is complex. Given the interchangeability of anxiety and depersonalisation, it is common for both states to occur in a client who appears for counselling and therapy. Though the former state may be recognised easily, the latter often remains unacknowledged in the counselling situation. This can lead to potential difficulties in the therapeutic relationship. For example, a poor response to relaxation methods may be incorrectly interpreted as a deliberate gesture of resistance by the therapist; in addition, complaints of lack of felt emotion may be interpreted as repression of feeling or an avoidance of spontaneity arising out of an overdeveloped superego, whereas this may not necessarily be the case. Depersonalisation and associated feelings of emotionlessness can arise from any stressful event whether it be intrapsychic or due to real external threat.

Bearing in mind the association between depersonalisation and arousal reduction, it is conceivable that some subjects will go through a depersonalised phase or complain of unreality feelings as anxiety diminishes. Therefore, we would speculatively suggest that a temporary state of depersonalisation, sometimes lasting several weeks, may hail the diminution of panic symptoms in much the same way as the state is an intrinsic part of rest following over-stimulation; as an intermediate stage of the change process, unreality feelings may legitimately be viewed as a favourable sign of progress, especially when they occur as long-standing neurotic problems are beginning to subside. For this reason, encouraging tolerance of the state can help in the transitional period, during which there is a shift towards a less stressful life style. If sufficient support and empathy is not given during this period, some individuals may inadvertently provoke further stress to alleviate the sense of detachment, a phenomenon amounting to a flight back into ill-health.

Nihilistic delusions

Depersonalisation has been frequently observed in depression. Delusions of nihil-
ism are common in severe depression and are likely to increase the level of
hopelessness and despair in such subjects. Nihilistic delusions reflect a sense of
loss of one's existence, and in depression these arise out of a conviction that the
world or the self has become lifeless and devoid of existence. Sims (1988) points
out that the ideation which accompanies depersonalisation is also nihilistic, though
to a less pronounced degree.

The pathogenesis of nihilistic delusions has been a subject of debate over the
years. It is possible that the superimposition of depersonalisation on a predominantly depressive picture may play a role. Subjects with primary depersonalisation
in the absence of clinical depression sometimes use analogies of non-existence
when they use the 'as if' prefix to describe their sensory impressions. An example
of this is a patient of one of the present authors, who described the experience of
the primary depersonalised state as feeling 'as if I wasn't part of myself, as if my
being had disappeared'. Another patient of one of the present authors, prone to
derealisation, described her sensory impressions of the world as follows: 'It's like
being in a void. My mind knows it's all around me [i.e. the occurrences of everyday
life events], but it seems as if it's fading away, like I'm in a sea of nothing and I
want to win it back. I cling to reality in case it disappears. It's as if I am falling into
a black hole of nothingness and never get back again'. The terms 'black hole' and
'void' are used by the patient as analogies to describe a lack of vividness of
perception, but, given the addition of an evaluation coloured by affective disorder,
the interpretation of dulled perception may be subtly changed. If the analogy of
emptiness of the external environment is dropped, so that the sensory impression
is interpreted as an actual diminution of external reality, the interpretation of these
perceptual changes may involve the conviction that reality itself is fading away.
This interpretation may account for the nihilistic cognitions common in a severe
depressive picture.

To emphasise this point, the above quote has been rewritten below, with the
prefixes indicating use of analogy placed in brackets. The patient's account then
reads as follows: 'It's [like] being in a void. My mind knows it's all around me, but
[it seems as if] it's fading away, [like] I'm in a sea of nothing and I want to win it
back. I cling to reality in case it disappears. [It's as if] I am falling into a black hole
of nothingness and never get back again'.

Whether the coexistence of depression alongside the depersonalised picture
leads to the abandonment of analogous thinking and the acceptance of cognitions
as literal fact is open to question. However, there is a striking resemblance between
nihilistic cognitions and cognitions which emanate from the depersonalised state
when the 'as if' qualifier is dropped.

Panic disorder

Fears of madness or dementia are common features of panic (Rachman and Maser 1988). It is interesting to note that fears of going mad or of dementing are also common in depersonalisation experiences. Though panic disorder patients are often preoccupied with somatic sensation, the emphasis which some panic patients place on fears of complete mental breakdown is more pronounced. It is feasible that at least some 'loss of consciousness fears' and 'loss of reasoning fears' are based on the impression of estrangement arising from a dysfunction of self-awareness.

Post-traumatic stress disorder

Marked depersonalisation is common in post-traumatic stress, and is a defining feature of PTSD as outlined by the DSM III classification system. Post-traumatic stress disorder is discussed in more detail elsewhere, but suffice it to say here that if PTSD is viewed as a perseveration of the reverberatory circuits signalling alarm, a reduction in awareness of feeling may serve the function of partial immunisation against overwhelming distress.

Depersonalisation is often prolonged and severe in post-traumatic stress, and may serve to insulate subjects from the intense feelings associated with the trauma itself. Flashbacks are common in post-traumatic stress, consisting of spontaneous, vivid images of the disturbing event, which is 'relived' during the flashback in the sense that patients describe the imagery and distress accompanying it as similar to that occurring during the initial trauma. It is probable that depersonalisation recedes during flashbacks, since patients describe flashback experiences as having intense felt-meaning; this intensity is contrary to the classical description of depersonalisation *per se.*

Sexual abuse

It has been acknowledged that sexual abuse may be regarded as precipitating post-traumatic stress. The experience of depersonalisation is common in adult subjects who have been sexually abused in childhood and there is evidence that, in some subjects, the depersonalised experience develops during the abuse itself, particularly when such events have been terrifying and repulsive. Some adult survivors are self-punitive in later life, and some clinicians and counsellors view self-punitive attitudes and behaviours as an attempt to alleviate guilt.

Self-mutilation

Slater and Roth (1969) reflect that the depersonalised individual often exhibits

> a quality of estrangement from and unfamiliarity with the self that makes the individual fearful or uncomfortable when left alone. He has feelings of doubt

about his identity. His reflection in the mirror appears unfamiliar and feelings of unreality may be heightened when he hears his own name spoken. He fears a sudden failure of memory, a lapse into blankness and total loss of identity. The physical experiences include feelings of floating into space and of blunted sensation all over the body which leads some patients to touch, punch or prick themselves repeatedly in an attempt to provoke a sense of reality.

(Slater and Roth 1969)

Some individuals who self-mutilate complain of unreality experiences when questioned closely about their general feeling-quality. There may be a volition towards self-harm of a physically-violent nature, in order to alleviate unreality feelings. Some self-mutilating patients prone to depersonalisation claim that by gaining the extra physical sensation arising out of pain, a sense of reality is achieved, associated with the acquisition of a vivid pain percept. There is likely to be a sensual aspect to the self-mutilation apart from the pain sensation and that peculiar sensation of subcutaneous intrusion; for example, the risk of permanent injury and serious harm may render self-experience more vivid by imparting a sense of urgency. Some self-mutilators, who never do themselves serious harm, are dismissed as 'attention-seekers' or 'hysterics', but may be compelled towards self-harm as a means of regaining a feeling of being-in-the-world, or the soma-belonging-to-me, by jolting themselves out of a sense of detachment.

DISCUSSION

Though early studies have linked depersonalisation with various forms of psychopathology, it is so commonplace that many normal people will experience it from time to time. When the unreality state is intense and prolonged, or occurs frequently, it can be distressing; in such cases, detailed phenomenological reflection with support and reassurance can be constructive. Some counsellors and therapists are sceptical of advocating states of tranquility as the universal antidote to distress as not all distressed individuals are over-aroused. Such scepticism seems particularly pertinent to therapeutic strategies with depersonalised subjects.

Moreover, it has been tentatively suggested that depersonalisation may occur at a transitional stage of counselling and therapy, coinciding with a general reduction of stress. If so, considerable support is necessary to prevent the new, unfamiliar, subjective experience from prompting the client back into a neurotic disposition. As resolution of psychological difficulties begins to occur, a sense of detachment can act as a useful holding device, giving time for adaptive emotional responses to take over from the prior maladaptive state.

In Chapter 3, we examined some of the evidence which suggests that distress and arousal do not co-vary perfectly; examples were given in which subjective anxiety peaks, without a corresponding elevation of physiological criteria in the direction traditionally assumed to correspond to the affect of fearfulness. Such findings have undermined the assumption that strategies of arousal reduction are a necessary component of the treatment of anxiety. It appears that in some instances, attempts at arousal reduction are inappropriate, since relaxation procedures have the result of increasing anxiety levels. This paradoxical effect, observed in a minority of patients, has been termed 'relaxation-induced anxiety'. The mechanisms underlying adverse reaction to relaxation-based techniques is as yet unclear, though a number of hypotheses have been considered recently. In some cases, described as 'relaxation-induced anxiety', it is clear that relaxation was not achieved at any stage of the process, since the relaxation procedure was interrupted by an anxiety reaction, at an early stage of its attempted application. In other cases, a state of relaxation was achieved, as defined by subjective and physiological criteria, before anxiety developed. The differentiation of clinical examples, based on the stage at which anxiety occurred during the relaxation procedure, is important; in some subjects, anxiety is almost certainly the product of the anticipated rather than actual effects of relaxation, while in others the relaxed state was achieved immediately prior to an anxiety bout.

Subjects who develop anxiety at the thought of relaxation are frequently apprehensive about losing control and have an inflated view of the potency of the relaxed state, particularly in generating or facilitating disinhibited or socially-embarrassing behaviour. Subjects whose anxiety is subsequent to the attainment of the relaxed state have experienced some of its consequences. These subjects typically report feeling distressed by the effects of relaxation itself, which they describe as unpleasant. In a sample of seven relaxed-induced-anxiety subjects who achieved a relaxed state immediately prior to anxiety, Fewtrell (1984/1986a) found that the development of fearfulness centred around disturbance of self-world relations. Complaints ranged from dizziness to sensations of estrangement and detachment, a state which one subject has described as 'being at sea in my own head'. If only to clarify the paradox of relaxation-induced anxiety, it is important to consider not only the possibility that high arousal is not an essential prerequisite of distress, but also the possibility that some states, characterised by low arousal, are aversive. One such state is depersonalisation.

There is no established treatment for depersonalisation. Various medical strategies have been applied, largely unsuccessfully, many of which were reviewed in an early paper by Davison (1964). Depersonalisation is a particularly interesting challenge to cognitive therapists. The problem differs from anxiety, panic disorder and depression, in that cognitive strategies for these are well established. There is an experimental literature on information-processing characteristics which accompany anxiety, depression and panic, but an absence of cognitive science literature on depersonalisation. Why, then, has depersonalisation been overlooked by cognitive research? The answer may lie in the nature of the problem, particularly the relation of self to body and self to world, which, as in severe depression, is not characterised by the negative meaning imposed upon events, but on the *absence* of meaning. Whereas cognitive approaches are adapted to the correction of interpretation of exteroceptive and interoceptive stimuli, which are experienced as vivid percepts or emotions, depersonalised patients exhibit an absence of vividness and some failure to appreciate self-participation in the experience itself.

SUMMARY

Not all distressing subjective states are associated with high autonomic arousal states, but conform to a pattern of low physiological output. Depersonalisation belongs to this category of problem, which possibly indicates an important feature in that, unlike the typical presentations of anxiety and panic disorder, interoceptive cues of raised cardiac output and increased respiration rate are unlikely to be present at the onset of a depersonalised episode; more research is badly needed in this area to clarify the sequence of internal events. The fact that relaxation approaches exacerbate the condition indicates that arousal reduction is largely unsuitable as a corrective strategy. However, cognitive approaches, which do not directly manipulate physiological activity, have not been tested.

The cognitions concomitant with depersonalisation include concern over the apparent inability to feel emotion and the impression that somatic sensation, thinking activity and the external world are somehow fading away, leading to such propositional statements as the commencement of madness, loss of the sensorium and imminent lapse into unconsciousness or oblivion. Patients yearn for the return of vivid sensation.

There is an established association between a number of psychopathological states and depersonalisation, including depression, post-traumatic stress disorder, self-injury and panic. It is suspected that some self-injury serves as an attempt to regain vivid sensation. Depersonalisation falls into the category of disorders which Jaspers (1963) terms 'disorders of awareness of activity'. Diminution in the feeling of one's own voluntary movement and thinking are particularly prominent in this disorder. Because disorders of awareness of activity are also present in the major psychoses, depersonalisation may provide a point of entry for cognitive psychologists to study this area of self-alienation, since depersonalised patients are usually co-operative and provide clear self-report data regarding their experiences of detachment.

Chapter 7

The psychopathology of craving

OVERVIEW OF CRAVING

The concept of craving is central to current conceptions of addictive behaviours and drug dependence. It is probable that if the concept of craving did not exist, it would be necessary to invent it to preserve the coherence of current models of drug use. The first problem we encounter is defining craving and measuring it. Craving is sometimes measured as a desire to use a psychoactive drug; a preference to use; an urge to use; a need to use. Some researchers suggest it is best measured subjectively, others biochemically or through accompanying physical signs and symptoms (e.g. West and Schneider 1987). Craving has been associated with a deprived physiological state, and so classified as an urge or drive of largely biochemical origin, over which the subject has little control. Conversely, among cognitivists craving is viewed increasingly as a self-induced thought state. A radical cognitive view would propose that craving is nothing other than the desire to ingest or otherwise experience the object of craving, and that the fluctuation of craving owes more to the rules of cognitive processing than to physiology.

The first part of this chapter reviews clinical evidence for and against these two opposed models of craving. In general, psychophysiological research does not support a one-to-one relation between the subjective reports of craving and physiological events. For example, intensity of craving is not necessarily proportional to indices of arousal. Furthermore, there is no consistent association between expressed craving and subsequent drug-use behaviour. But physiology is not irrelevant to the desire to use drugs and there are identifiable changes in physiological measures prior to use, though these changes are variable across subjects. While the onset of craving can sometimes have an impulsive quality, it can also accumulate incrementally. It may start as a thought, or as a feeling-sensation, which elicits propositional thoughts that are held with considerable conviction. By changing the focus of thoughts, or by challenging their content, the craver can influence craving; however, the results of such clinical intervention are inconsistent. The craving urge can also be qualitatively modified by factors such as current social context, interpersonal relations, motor behaviour and physiological state, in a way which is not easily explained by a purely cognitive model. Although some craving is episodic and can appear or disappear abruptly from the consciousness of the user, other types of craving are embedded in the everyday ebb and flow of awareness. Here, craving predictably accompanies other coping difficulties. In such cases, craving may be considered as part of a style of coping with a difficult situation rather than the result of a drug-induced chemical deprivation. The psychological 'acts' which occur immediately before and after the 'act' of craving do not necessarily form a consistent pattern and the intentional object of craving – the object towards which the act of craving is directed – is not always drug use.

The latter part of this chapter suggests that craving is an 'act' in its own right; a qualitatively distinct series of preparatory states. These preparatory states have contributing cognitive, feeling-state and physiological components, and the cognitive element is not necessarily in control. These preparatory states are self-contained 'acts' and not tied to subsequent behaviour; nor is the form of craving specific to the substance abused. Craving represents a mode of being in the world peculiar to the person rather than to blanket pharmacological or cognitive factors. A phenomenological approach can help identify personal elements which are clinically useful in modifying these preparatory states.

PHYSIOLOGICAL ACCOUNTS OF CRAVING

The simplest model of craving is that it closely relates to absence of drug use. Therefore, though the effects of drugs vary widely, craving always has the same purpose, to motivate drug use. As Miller and Gold put it: 'Addiction implies a loss of control over the use of [benzodiazepines] supported by a drive to use, which probably has a neurochemical basis located in the limbic system' (1990: 24). Or as Tiffany says: 'In all theories urges and cravings are seen as the primary determinants of ongoing drug-use behavior in addicts and as the principal cause of relapse in addicts attempting abstinence' (1990: 150). Shiffman's statement that 'the urge to smoke when it becomes stronger than the ex-smoker's determination to quit leads to relapse' (1979: 158) summarises this prevalent view.

Current neurochemical theories of craving do not suggest a direct link between physiological state and craving behaviour, but propose that this link is mediated by some form of conditioned association. The physiological deprivation is thus cued via another signal system, which has better access to conscious behaviour. This link may be internal or external. So, for example, the opponent-process theory of Solomon and Corbit (1973) sees the effects of drugs tied to stimulation of the brain-reward centres, and therefore the user initially takes drugs for pleasure. A conscious association builds up between pleasure and drug taking. But later on, as drug tolerance develops, the person ingests more of the substance to avoid the discomfort produced by the drug-deprived homeostatic corrections that have disturbed normal levels of functioning. Craving is the reaction to the loss of pleasurable associations.

An alternative view, presented by Siegel (1983), is that drug effects are associated with the environment in which they are taken. So, environmental signals elicit what Siegel terms 'a drug-compensatory conditioned response' (CR) that adjusts the body to the drug effect. This CR produces craving in the presence of situational stimuli. Hence, an organism is at risk of overdosing when the drug is administered in an environment that has not been previously paired with the drug (and thus does not elicit the compensatory pharmacological CR that attenuates the effect of the drug).

There seem to be three separate but entangled physiologies to consider in clarifying the role of craving in drug use:

1   the physiology of drug effects
2   the physiology of drug withdrawal
3   the physiology of craving.

The physiological model would predict a systematic relationship between the criteria exhibited during each stage, particularly that the effects of withdrawal would match the effects of craving. Unfortunately, there is little correlation either between or within these distinct effects. The empirical findings are in this respect parallel to physiological studies of anxiety and panic, in that neither changes in physiological quality nor amplitude portray a consistent psychological equivalence (Beck 1988). The same physiological effects can produce paradoxical subjective reports. For example, a standardised dose of nicotine produces a feeling of calm in some smokers but arouses others (D. J. Gilbert 1979).

Drug-induced physiological changes are well documented. For example the effect of nicotine administered in moderate doses is to increase heart-rate, stimulate catecholamines and increase motor reactivity. The effect of cocaine is to produce increases in systolic and diastolic blood pressure and heart-rate, and cortical excitation. Motor and respiratory factors show little change. The effect of benzodiazepines is on GABA-ergic pathways and produces depression of the CNS, somnolence, motor incoordination and disinhibiting effects. Amphetamine is primarily a psychomotor stimulant, but can also produce racing thoughts and tremulousness. Caffeine is generally regarded as a CNS stimulant, but in heavy doses produces symptoms indistinguishable from anxiety (nervousness, insomnia, sensory disturbances, agitation and activation of peripheral arousal measures). These effects are generally uniform across subjects, though their intensity may be modified behaviourally (Janke 1978 for review). The pre-ingestion metabolic state of the person may mitigate or augment the effects.

The physiological effects of the ingested substance are known to vary according to a number of factors, including quantity and rate of ingestion. Ingestion patterns vary widely between subjects, and as soon as we introduce self-administration into the equation the physiological effects show correspondingly wider individual differences than when supervised ingestion is regulated and standardised. During smoking, acceleration of heart-rate varies according to smoking strategy. Response to task demand also varies across individual smokers (O'Connor 1992). The introverted smoker uses tobacco very differently from an extrovert during a stressful vigilance task (Eysenck 1980). The effects of psychoactive drugs may be attenuated or augmented depending on the environment and social setting in which they are taken (Henningfield *et al.* 1991).

A distinction must be made between patients self-administering the drug for euphoric purposes and those patients or animals receiving the drug in an ahedonic, medical context. Patients who receive morphine, for example, unconsciously are far less likely to develop a dependence than following recreational use, and when introduced as a temporary palliative, the drug may be phased out, usually with no adverse reports other than constipation and lack of sexual appetite (Bejerot 1984).

Though the physiological effects of drugs tend to be receptor-specific to the drug in question, the effects of cessation of ingestion are diverse. The withdrawal effects of caffeine may include headaches, anxiety, increased muscle tension, muscle pains and lethargy, but there may also be beneficial effects, such as reductions in tachycardia, hypertension and gastro-intestinal complaints (Rizzo *et al.* 1988). However, there are some widely observed withdrawal effects assumed to be specific to each drug type. Opiate withdrawal is said to involve 'a host of painful sensations, intolerable feelings, oppressive organic disturbances of every sort, combined with an extreme psychic excitement, intense restlessness and persistent insomnia' (Lindesmith 1984: 34). The withdrawal symptoms most associated with not smoking are: irritability, hunger, depression, poor concentration, restlessness (Shiffman 1979; Hughes *et al.* 1989). The effects of alcohol withdrawal include: pulse racing, tremor, sweating, agitation, insomnia, lowered sex drive and depression. Withdrawal symptoms associated with benzodiazepines include: paresthesia, numbness, tremors, muscle stiffness, myalgia. Headache is common and gastro-intestinal symptoms may include nausea, vomiting, constipation and diarrhoea. Cardiovascular symptoms may include palpitations, chest pain, hyperventilation and malaise.

The existence of withdrawal symptoms would strengthen the argument in favour of a chemical basis of craving if: the effects of withdrawal are indeed closely related to the specific actions of the drug in question; there is a direct link between severity of drug use and severity of withdrawal symptoms; the effects of withdrawal are eliminated by drug use and by no other means. However, withdrawal symptoms are notoriously variable both within and between individuals. Miller and Gold (1990) note that the manifestations of withdrawal from benzodiazepines (BZD) show a broad spectrum of signs and symptoms, which occur in varying frequency and severity. The more common signs of BZD withdrawal, such as anxiety, hyperactivity and agoraphobia, insomnia and depression, are similar in form to withdrawal from alcohol and other sedative-hypnotic drugs. Furthermore, many of the symptoms, such as sleepiness and hyperactivity, are clearly mutually exclusive and this emphasises the point that there are wide individual differences in the experience.

The anxiety following BZD withdrawal is often indistinguishable from the anxiety disorders for which BZD was originally employed. In other words, the withdrawal may simply indicate a resurgence of the original problem. Tobacco withdrawal often mimics grief or other emotional reactions, and the severity of withdrawal is a function of personality and the personal stress experienced by the person at the time and manner of cessation (Bliss *et al.* 1989). Pomerleau and Pomerleau (1988) note the variability of withdrawal leaves its chemical basis uncertain. Peele (1985) in his review concludes that modern models of addiction have consistently overestimated the amount of variance in addiction accounted for by the chemical properties of specific substances.

Tyrer *et al.* (1983) studied withdrawal reactions in thirty-six out-patients who had been taking benzodiazepines for six months or longer. All patients were converted to a standard dose of diazepam, and were then withdrawn completely over a 28-day period. An interesting feature of this study is that all the subjects were withdrawn from the active agent without their knowledge, owing to the use of a placebo to supplement the regime. The design of the study enabled a discrimination between actual but surreptitious withdrawal and pseudo-withdrawal, in which the same subjects were led to believe they were withdrawing, but were in fact progressively being weaned off their placebo. The magnitude of distress, as defined by the CPRS (Asberg *et al.* 1978), was greater following actual withdrawal than following pseudo-withdrawal for every symptom-frequency quoted. In particular, actual withdrawal was associated with a markedly higher frequency of transient sleep disturbance, appetite reduction, sadness and depersonalisation phenomena than was found in pseudo-withdrawal. Nonetheless, pseudo-withdrawal also had a demonstrably adverse effect. Tyrer *et al.*'s data suggest that recovery from actual withdrawal takes approximately six weeks, with a continuing trend of improvement to below the pre-withdrawal baseline at follow-up three to five months later.

Higgit *et al.* (1985) suggest that the rate of dosage reduction should depend on the withdrawal symptoms in the individual case and should be titrated accordingly. Tyrer *et al.* (1983) observed true withdrawal symptoms in only half of their subjects, the other half showing no apparent ill-effects. They searched for factors which might discriminate between the two groups and found that withdrawal reaction was unrelated to dosage level at the time of withdrawal; neither was it related to a fall in serum nor diazepam, duration of drug treatment (conflicting with the findings of Hallstrom and Lader 1982), or age and gender of the subjects. The only predictive factor was personality, as defined by the Personality Assessment Schedule, or PAS (Tyrer and Alexander 1979), which was administered to an informant close to the patient at the start of the study. Problematic withdrawers were significantly more likely to score high on passive-dependence and anankastic traits, but not on schizoid, sociopathic or dysthymic traits. It is interesting that dysthymia is a personality factor which, according to Tyrer and Alexander (1979), is loaded by 'anxiousness'.

A word of caution should be provided when dealing with tranquilliser-dependent patients. Golombok *et al.* (1987) followed up a series of patients, who had undergone withdrawal, for a period of five years, a considerably longer follow-up period than in most other studies. At the end of the five years, continued abstinence was only 54 per cent, and 60 per cent of the subjects showed a significant degree of psychiatric disturbance, as defined by GHQ scores. The authors conclude that a medical approach to withdrawal is therefore insufficient and needs to be supplemented by 'psychological adjuncts' to prevent relapse. Success in withdrawal is influenced by the amount and quality of support available at the time of withdrawal. Stopforth (1986) has recommended the introduction of a behavioural approach to anxiety management to bolster coping skills prior to withdrawal, followed by attendance at a support group during and following the withdrawal period itself. One such procedure could be adapted from that provided by Archer and Reisor (1982), which is described with sufficient clarity to be replicated.

The diagnostic term 'dependence', as used in a nosology of substance-dependence disorders in DSM-III-R (APA 1987), does not require withdrawal syndrome as a necessary defining criterion. Withdrawal symptoms include a variety of factors, the origin of which cannot simply be chemical readjustment. There is also an emotional component, which includes symptoms such as anxiety or depression. Moreover, the overlap of effects across different drug withdrawals suggests that substances share some common withdrawal effects. It would appear that the longer the time since cessation of ingestion, the greater the convergence of withdrawal features. Drug-specific features tend to disappear after the first few days of detoxification.

The consequences of cessation of ingestion are generally reported in the literature as negative affect states. There is little mention of the positive effects of withdrawal, such as the greater acuity, confidence, and clear-headedness frequently reported by ex-smokers (O'Connor and Langlois 1991). It is as though most practitioners *expect* or *assume* that withdrawal must be a negative experience. The chemical view of craving would consider the physiology of withdrawal as an alarm system that triggers desire when the body's demands are not met. This means withdrawal is viewed as a passive response to absence of the drug. It therefore follows that there should be a strong link between craving and somatic signs of withdrawal. Tiffany (1990), in a review, indicates very low correlations between physiological variables and self-reported urges toward continued consumption. Tiffany notes that the overall magnitude of correlations between physiological response and craving was not impressive. The average of all correlations accounted for less than 15 per cent of the variance. Even when the analysis was restricted to the ten significant correlations, the average accounted for approximately 27 per cent of the variance. In some cases in this review coefficients were not reported, but investigators explicitly stated that they were not significant. Tiffany concludes that these low correlations are particularly troublesome for some craving theories (e.g. Ludwig and Wikler 1974; Siegel 1983), which claim that conditioned physiological responses provide the source of craving.

Tiffany also reviewed studies comparing withdrawal-related craving and recidivism. The average correlation between craving and subsequent use across nine studies was 0.40, accounting for 16 per cent of the variance. Hughes *et al.* (1989) found no relationship between withdrawal severity, abstinence discomfort and recidivism. Both Stitzer and Gross (1988) and West *et al.* (1989) found a lack of association between withdrawal severity and abstinence following the first few days of cessation. Interestingly, though Stitzer and Gross (1988) found no relationship between withdrawal severity and subsequent relapses, they still argued that there *must* still be a strong presumptive link!!

In the cigarette-cessation literature treatments, such as nicotine chewing gum or patches, that rely on the idea of reducing withdrawal symptoms for their rationale are no more successful than other (cognitive-behavioural) programmes and may be less so if not combined with supplementary counselling. Furthermore, phasing out cigarettes gradually is no more successful than abrupt cessation (Brown *et al.* 1984). The ecological basis of much craving suggests that improving coping skills, restructuring the environment and social support may be more pertinent in preventing relapse than focusing on withdrawal (Ginsberg *et al.* 1992).

In summary, the three hypotheses of the chemical model of craving remain unsupported in that:

1 chronic withdrawal symptoms are not specific to drugs
2 the intensity of these effects is not related to subsequent use
3 craving is not uniquely alleviated by treatments aimed at abating withdrawal symptoms.

An additional point noted clinically by Marlatt and Gordon (1985) concerns the tendency of ex-users to attribute difficult experiences, which are unrelated to substance ingestion, to feelings caused by withdrawal. For example, a clinically-depressed patient may falsely attribute concentration problems to the lack of sufficient cigarettes, or coffee.

Craving, by definition, requires self-reflection, which can therefore be reported. It is unclear whether desire or approach behaviours show *greater* situational specificity; most questionnaires assessing desire or preference to use a drug show a more robust factor-analytic situational structure than that for actual ingestion behaviour. However, cigarette or alcohol *use* may be automatic, occasioned by ritual or social pressure, and only on occasion be a result of individual-centred volition. In other words, some subjects often use drugs without first craving them. Craving sometimes begins at the point at which the user decides to use rather than prior to use. In other words, *the act of approach induces craving*. This aspect is represented clinically in several reports of smokers and drinkers who only crave after they have thought of the cigarette or drink (see Marlatt 1985). Craving may therefore precede an approach orientation, or may follow the cues of approach, or, for that matter, ingestion. A person who eats, say, a chocolate because it is offered may subsequently crave more despite the initial absence of appetitive activity.

Mood may be one mediating element in deciding the temporal sequence of craving and use. There is some evidence that craving prior to use may be linked with depressive feelings and that the reporting of somatic sensations of withdrawal is more likely under negative than positive emotional states (Kozlowski and Heatherton 1990). People immersed in negative affect are likely to experience withdrawal more intensely and are more likely to report it. Craving after use, however, may be more a consequence of positive mood; smoking for example, may produce enjoyment and promote the desire to repeat the behaviour. Craving after use here is more at a cognitive level of preference. But this point needs to be further explored.

Withdrawal symptoms, like any aversive state, are likely to lead to attempts to alleviate them, but this will not necessarily lead to drug use. It may lead to the contrary, a deliberate strategy to inhibit drug use. Whether the experience of withdrawal leads to use depends on support network, environment, self-efficacy, and alternative coping strategies. Siegel (1983) makes the point that we should distinguish between acute withdrawal symptoms, which are the result of feedback systems, and the feed-forward mechanisms, which produce anticipation of effects. The latter are drug-compensatory conditioned responses and may be more usefully termed 'preparation' rather than 'withdrawal' symptoms. Siegel argues that the conditioned responses (CRs) are the person's way of preparing for the effects of the drug by producing the opposite effects to the drug. These preparation symptoms can be elicited by any associated cues, including cognitive cues, or situational demand (Woodson *et al.* 1983). An addict returning to his/her neighbourhood may display withdrawal which is absent in novel settings. Drug-associated stimuli, such as needles, or friends or cafés or even sounds, can elicit withdrawal preparation.

Siegel's theory refers mainly to physiological aspects of withdrawal, and he originally suggested CRs were always in the opposite direction to drug effects. However, this is not so, and physiological reactions prior to drug use can be in any direction. More recently, Siegel *et al.* (1988) have suggested that when UCS-elicited activities are afferent and involve sensory effects the CR will be in the same direction as the drug effect. When they have an efferent site of action and elicit motor activity then the CR will be in the opposite direction. But it is not easy to sort out which is which, and Siegel concludes vaguely: 'In the case of those drugs with multiple effects, the various components of the CR would be expected to mimic or mirror the drug effect, depending on the mechanism by which the effect results' (Siegel *et al.* 1988). We might also ask how he accounts for the times when there are no related physiological accompaniments to craving and where desire is at the level of a cognitive choice or preference. Most of Siegel's work is conducted in a laboratory environment where a preparatory effect may well be conditioned in isolation. But in reality, other factors, such as the movement involved in lighting up a cigarette, may produce 'effects' equal or greater to the autonomic conditioning, and often movement and conditioned effects cannot be separated.

However, if we retain Siegel's feed-forward idea and consider that the physiology of craving reflects primarily an active preparatory state, it may be that these preparatory states are part of the support physiology required effectively to carry out the task in hand and not just preparation for the cigarette. In other words, before a vigilance task the person may prepare for a cigarette in a different manner than after eating a meal, because the task demands are different. The state of craving is linked with anticipation of task demand rather than just anticipation of drug reaction. O'Connor (1989a) has reviewed evidence suggesting that motor preparation influences the desire to smoke and the subsequent effects of smoking.

To conclude, there is no doubt that drugs have physiological effects; when the drugs are injected or administered directly to the CNS, the effects are generally uniform and the subjective effects to a greater or lesser degree also uniform; but as soon as the drug is self-administered the effects become more variable, depending on what the person is doing, on personality, on their expectations and social situation. Withdrawal effects are even more variable and non-specific and it is not clear which are the effects of the drugs, which are emotional cues, and which are products of arousal states induced by situational factors of stress (since withdrawal is more likely to be experienced under stress anyway). Very acute withdrawal symptoms are pharmacologically cued and usually last a matter of days, but thereafter the physiological cues seem situationally cued, either by conditioning or by cognitive factors of expectancy. What seems clear is that craving, far from being a product of *feedback* from pharmacological actions, is a *feed-forward* mechanism actively preparing the craver either, as Siegel suggests, for the drug effects or, as O'Connor proposes, for situational demands surrounding the drug use. Discussion of preparation brings us to expectancies, and into the cognitive aspects of desire to use. Craving from a cognitive point of view includes time spent thinking about the drug, deliberating on the strength of urge to use, expected benefits from drug use and confidence in not using.

COGNITIVE MODELS OF CRAVING

A number of studies have shown that positive beliefs and expectations about drug use promote desire to use. Leigh (1989), for example, studied the predictability of drinking attitudes on subsequent drinking behaviour. She found that positive expectancies both of the physical and social effects of drinking predicted quantity consumed, but that overall attitude towards adult drinking was a more important predictor of general drinking behaviour.

Clinically speaking, cognitive techniques have now been employed in all areas of cessation. Beck-style Socratic dialogues and questioning pros and cons to continuing a habit, challenging expectations and aiding decision-making are routine in drug-dependency clinics. Cognitive techniques used specifically to cope with craving include distraction techniques, thought-stopping and imagery. Drug users are able quite literally to put craving out of their mind, for example, when it is accepted that there is no possibility of smoking in a no-smoking office. Craving is a reflective state and this is highlighted by the change in consciousness that can distance a person from their craving. Marlatt *et al.* (1985) describe a variety of such distancing techniques using the 'Samurai' or 'bouncing ball' method, whereby subjects imagine their craving going up and down like a ball, or being cut down like a Samurai. Imagery and narrative can also have the same effect. A person can reduce desire to use by changing their focus from a positive to a negative expectation, but this reduction is only temporary.

It is not clear how successful cognitive techniques by themselves are at eradicating either craving or subsequent substance use without the help of behavioural strategies such as exposure, or situational coping skills (Heather and Bradley 1990). Leigh (1989) concludes that although investigators assume that expectancies influence behaviour, behaviour may instead influence expectancies, and the best predictor of future habits may be past habits rather than past thoughts. Young *et al.* (1990) also report that although alcohol-related expectancies remain stable over situations, the influence expectancies exert on actual drinking is not known. O'Connor and Langlois (1993) compared a purely cognitive treatment aimed at raising self-efficacy with a behavioural treatment package for smokers at high risk of relapse. They found both craving and efficacy improved more in the behavioural group, and that cognitive strategies developed in the behavioural group more spontaneously than did behavioural strategies in the cognitive group.

Cognitive techniques are particularly useful in motivating a person to stop using, and are of help in relapse prevention. Typically, in the early stages of non-use, cognitive methods must be combined with behavioural strategies for maximum efficacy and it is not conclusive that cognitive factors alone are responsible for changes in degree of desire (MacKay and Marlatt 1990–1991). Awareness by the addict of the situational character and potential controllability of desire to use can itself be a factor in diminishing the importance of craving and raising confidence in coping with desire to use (O'Connor and Physant-Skov 1989). Minneker-Hügel *et al.* (1992) concluded, from their comparative study of relapse in groups of smokers receiving and not receiving structured relapse prevention, that long-term self-observation of smoking extending beyond the period of cessation has a better chance of lowering relapse rate than prevention training within the therapy period.

For a cognitive model to be sound it must be able to show that:

(a) the source of craving is a self-persuasive thought state resulting from faulty expectations, self-statement, or other cognitive misprocessing;
(b) craving can be modified by thought processes more than by other interventions;
(c) there is an identifiable pattern of cognitions associated with craving.

Unlike the pharmacological model, there is no coherent cognitive model of craving. The cognitive attempts to explain craving fall into two categories, namely: attribution approaches and skills approaches. An attributional perspective, along the lines of Schachter and Singer's (1962) thesis, would approach the problem in terms of the evaluation of sensation. In this theoretical context, craving represents a process whereby physiological cues are interpreted as negatively hedonic, prompting the desire to use in order to obtain an improved feeling state. Emphasis may be given to the evaluation of drug-induced somatic changes which are perceived by the user to indicate well-being, so that different interpretations, such as personal repercussions, are assessed more objectively.

The attribution model assumes that correcting attributions should take away desire by itself. However, information and re-attribution regarding physiological sensations does not help deal with craving. The most successful cognitive strategies appear to be distraction, redefining positive expectancies, rehearsing self-statements, and awareness, not re-attribution of withdrawal symptoms or drug effects.

Attributions may, however, be indirectly affected by other procedures (Peele 1985). Attributing a positive social image to smoking, such as construing the behaviour as sophisticated or glamorous, are poor prognostic factors of quitting (O'Connor and Stravynski 1982; Owen and Brown 1991). Available evidence suggests, contrary to the attribution model, that drug users narrow their somatic focus during use and ignore intruding physical sensations (Callaway *et al.* 1992; Hansen *et al.* 1989).

The social learning or adaptational model is that adopted by Marlatt (1985), who tends to view craving as a continuous process of social-self-management. The person adapts to drugs because the alternatives are worse. The user has problems adapting to the environment, for example, a maturity problem, a familial problem or a self-esteem problem. Craving springs from a yearning to fit in, and from a failure to cope, which the user projects the onto the 'substitute adaptation' of drug use. Marlatt views continued use as related largely to restricted self-expectancies, low self-efficacy, negative metaphors, and unsuccessful coping with life. Enforcing non-use requires changing the person's life style, the way the person perceives the drug, and their ability to cope with life and, in particular, how the person deals with abstinence-violation effects. This social-learning model is frequently employed as a relapse-prevention model, though in practice it mixes strategies and it is not clear what components are more essential, cognitive or behavioural self-management (e.g. Curry *et al.* 1988; Havassy *et al.* 1991; Minneker-Hügel *et al.* 1992). The adaptational or social-learning approach has so far offered a model of how to manage cognitions associated with use or non-use, rather than a cognitive explanation of craving.

Tiffany (1990) in his cognitive-skill model proposes that craving can be conceptualised as responses supported by non-automatic processing that are activated in parallel with drug-use schemata. According to this cognitive model, there are two major situations under which non-automatic processing might be invoked: (a) some environmental condition impedes or blocks the drug-use action plan in an individual not attempting to avoid drug use, or (b) non-automatic cognitive processes are invoked in an explicit attempt to impede or block a drug-use action plan. There should be a fundamental difference between the non-automatic processing elicited by these two types of situation. In the first situation, non-automatic processes are activated in support of drug use, in the second, to counteract drug use.

Tiffany's (1990) basic idea is that drug behaviour is automatic while craving is a conscious reflection on this behaviour, so craving will arrive at times in the drug behaviour where difficulties are encountered and actions are no longer automatic. According to Tiffany, the cognitions and support physiology surrounding craving are either related to the effort to facilitate abstinence or to avoid abstinence. He suggests that very distinct cognitions are attached to the different modes of craving. Desire to use is associated with thoughts about obtaining the drug; desire not to use is paired with ideas of how to avoid the drug. In further laboratory experiments Tiffany reports that imagery which elicits craving also elicits appropriate changes in support physiology (Tiffany and Hakenewerth 1991).

According to Tiffany, craving includes distinct cognitive conceptualisations, such as desire to smoke, intention to smoke, anticipation of outcome from smoking, anticipation of relief from negative emotion, and each of these will vary depending on the purpose of craving. The clinical implication of Tiffany's model is that retraining the user in the skill of preparing to inhibit use by means of text or imagery should change the nature of craving.

A major problem with Tiffany's model is that it relies heavily on the distinction between automatic and controlled processing; in reality, no act can be either one or the other. Craving as a thought process involves both habitual and controlled components as does drug behaviour, hence neither one is entirely automatic or controlled. Another problem is that expressions of craving are much more diverse than Tiffany's model would allow. Although conscious thoughts at a certain point in the craving cycle may be categorised according to whether they concern getting the drug or not getting it, other thoughts revolve around specific events related to flow of behaviour and do not necessarily express monolithic or binary (either/or) intention. Also, in Tiffany's model, as in all cognitive models, preference is given to cognitive self-schema in orchestrating craving, when the situational cues could just as easily operate through activating somatic adaptation or sensorial schemata. Smells or sounds can elicit craving and Tiffany's cognitive categorisation of self-reported desire does not do justice to the way craving fits in with the flow of experience.

Above all, the cognitive position introduces a subtle level of situational analysis of craving. The cognitive position provides compelling reasons to consider cognitions associated with craving and drug effects as independent. The motivational aspects of craving do not necessarily relate well to the effects of the drug and so it is not surprising that, for example, smokers crave a cigarette only to extinguish it after lighting up because the effects are not pleasant. Cocaine users, for example, frequently anticipate positive 'highs' from use, whereas after use they routinely report dysphoria (Resnick and Resnick 1984). Craving is an independent preparatory state not conditioned to drug effects. Cognitive evidence suggests that craving is not a mechanistic product of pharmacological factors, but an active preparation towards an anticipated state.

Anticipation is, of course, a propositional cognitive process, but may be influenced more immediately by concurrent motor activity than by thoughts. O'Connor (1989a) suggested that it is useful to dichotomise the craving for cigarettes into two mutually-exclusive situational categories, namely, when the person was actively engaged in a task and when they were not. These two states invoke different inhalation patterns and produce different effects on the smoker. This typing on the basis of background behavioural activity has clinical implications, since those who smoke when engaged tend to benefit more from situationally-based reduction of use than do those who prefer to smoke when not engaged (O'Connor and Langlois 1993).

The level of background activity during smoking itself offers a valid categorisation of smokers, since there are motivational differences between those who smoke under high or low activity levels. These differences have been shown to relate both to long-term differences in action set and to phasic differences in event-related motor preparation (O'Connor 1989a). Those who smoke during skilled tasks which involve concentration employ cigarettes differently from those who smoke to alleviate boredom. In an attentional task, smoking gates out distraction (Knott 1985) and forms a task secondary to attention. In a low-activity task associated with boredom, smoking improves mood and acts as a primary task. Smoking also interacts as a skill with the skill level on the primary task. Some smokers smoke more in unskilled attentional situations (including most laboratory situations) than in skilled ones. In the unskilled case, smoking during concentration may help to reduce spare degrees of freedom that arise from dual task difficulties (Abernethy 1988). In the skilled case, smoking will, on the contrary, create unwanted degrees of freedom and so itself become a distractor.

A QUALITATIVE TAXONOMY OF CRAVING

Craving represents an anticipation of, or desire for, a state not yet achieved. It is an experience in itself, and can be compartmentalised as conceptually separate from the craved object, such as a cigarette, or the state springing from the effect of such an object. The context of the preparatory act of craving begins and ends with other activities being planned at the same time. A person anticipates finishing work. A scenario is evoked by this anticipation including thoughts of leaving work, relaxing, smoking a cigarette, driving home, meeting with spouse. This preparatory plan is reinforced by a number of actions, for example, self-statements and self-persuasive thoughts made by the person. The intentional object of craving is to forward this preparatory cycle, of which anticipating a cigarette is part, along with anticipating relaxing and leaving work. The person craves a cigarette in the context of preparing for a range of other activities evoked by the preparation scenario. Consequently, a number of events besides the thought of the cigarette may change the nature of craving were, for example, the person to work late, or discover a reason to change the plan to go home. Since there is a general anticipation of events, in which craving for a cigarette, as one event, is embedded, changes in these accompanying events, for example, going home, relaxing or finishing work, may also change craving. In clinical experience it is not uncommon for craving to disappear with an abrupt change of task demand. A nurse craving a cigarette in her office forgets about it when called outside; similarly, a journalist assigned an easy story to write when she was expecting a difficult one experiences a decrease in craving.

Cognitive narrative plays a large part in defining the unit of craving, since it is with self-talk that the person conjures up and maintains a credible sequence, a middle and an end of the anticipation. All of which is expressed and fed back verbally to reinforce preparatory thoughts and actions, constituting the preparatory state. Marlatt (1985) has alluded to the importance of narrative and metaphor in smokers' accounts of their habit, and in maintaining beliefs about its inevitability. Of course, whenever the preparatory unit comes to an end, another preparation is initiated and so another self-contained preparatory act commences. It follows that the comparison unit for craving is not to be found from comparing cigarette effects (i.e. adjacent acts), but by looking for family resemblances among similar preparatory incidents sharing similar intentionality. By comparing similar preparatory acts, the person's style of preparation rather than the single element of craving itself is identified as the relevant context to address in intervention.

Some sample quotes taken from cigarette smokers convey the diversity of cognitive influences associated with craving:

(a) I light up just like that without thinking. Suddenly I find a cigarette in my hand.

(b) I was chatting with friends late at night and we ran out of cigarettes, I felt this need for a smoke, I went round the streets looking for a machine. I lit it up but put it out after a few puffs, I didn't seem to want it any more.

(c) I always have it mind that I will light up a cigarette when I've finished the job – during break – so I'm really expecting it. By the time break comes I'm really craving.

(d) I can't do any writing without a cigarette. I can't concentrate without a cigarette, it's the one time I can't do without.

(e) The craving is definitely physical with me. I start aching for a cigarette. I feel it in the pit of my stomach and at the back of my throat. It's really out of my control.

(f) I find it easy not to smoke in front of my kids. I just decided I wouldn't and that was it. I don't even consider it anymore.

(g) When I'm in a meeting I accept I can't smoke, I don't even think about it. But when the meeting's over I'm dying for a smoke as soon as I get out.

(h) I can smoke or not smoke. If I've got nothing to do I'll smoke and enjoy it. If I'm busy I don't bother. It doesn't worry me one way or another.

(i) I was about to light up in the ward office and this patient starts yelling, so we had to deal with that for about 30 minutes. I'd clean forgotten about the cigarette. Then I saw it in the ashtray and the craving was back.

(j) I can't say I enjoy smoking, it's definitely a habit with me, but I miss it if I don't smoke. I get irritable. My husband says – you better have a smoke – so I have one.

(k) After an argument, I just smoke one after another, it's emotional really – calms me down, gives me somewhere to direct my energy.

So we see that the smoker may experience craving as: intense or non-existent, external or internal. Craving may be satisfied by smoking or not satisfied by smoking; it may be temporary or long term; emotional or cognitive; controllable or uncontrollable; an antecedent to one event or a consequence of another event. Each of these poles is represented in the statements listed previously, and its meaning can be located in whatever 'act' the person is preparing to do and the style in which they are preparing it. So, looking descriptively at craving, we can say that craving is not a uniform experience and is not tied to a specific drug effect. Craving is effectively a function of personal coping style.

CRAVING AND PERSONAL STYLE

Both drug use and intensity of craving have been tied with personality and general life-style factors. Factors such as impulsiveness, sensation-seeking and the Pd scale of the MMPI, plus a variety of ego dysfunction and dysfunctional family conditions have been associated with dependence (see Peele 1985 for a review). As Robins (1984) has pointed out, the stereotype of the heroin addict as someone with a monomaniacal craving for a single drug seems hardly accurate since heroin users also use other drugs regularly. There are clear connections between drug use and other life-style factors in all drug users.

Ninety percent of alcoholics also smoke. A majority of BZD users drink too much. Mechanic (1979) found smokers were less likely to wear seat belts, while Kalant and Kalant (1976) found users of both prescribed and illicit amphetamines suffered more accidents. Smokers have 40 per cent higher accident rates than non-smokers (McGuire 1972) and tend to have a whole gamut of negative health habits and health expectancies and stress coping styles (evasion, procrastination), and low self-efficacy.

Substance-abuse disorders also commonly overlap with other conditions, such as anxiety, depression and sociopathy. Zucker and Gomberg (1986) identified several specific pre-morbid factors associated with increased likelihood of poor treatment outcome in alcoholism: anti-social behaviour, poor school achievement, hyperactivity, poor or superficial interpersonal relations, parental or marital conflict. But whereas drug use and relapse can be predicted from general personality and social factors, intensity of craving seems to relate more to individualised and situation-specific coping styles.

Khantzian (1984) notes that 'narcissistic' vulnerabilities are predisposing factors to high craving, coupled with special problems in accepting emotional dependencies and in actively acknowledging and pursuing goals and satisfactions related to needs and wants. Prominent defences and traits include extreme repression, disavowal, self-sufficiency, alternation of solicitous and angry demands, and an unstable and chaotic organisation, which invites limit-setting but then fights against it. Many addicts were abused as children and the feeling of helplessness leads to the search for a strong external protector. Most of the studies comparing strength of desire to use, pathology and personal style have been psychodynamic. However, current rather than historical data may be more pertinent to a pragmatic formulation.

O'Connor and Bradley (1990) report the case of an amphetamine user who craved when she felt unable to cope with the demands to which she was exposed. On further investigation, her cognitive structure contained a number of classic suppositions outlined by Beck and Emery (1985) as typical of depressives, such as:

a   low self-confidence, 'I'm not really any good';
b   low sense of control over life, 'I feel like I'm on a conveyor belt';
c   poor self-identity, 'never feel I am being my real self'.

These cognitive elements were the targets of intervention.

A descriptive account of craving would shift attention away from antecedent and consequent 'effects' towards analysis of personal classes of consciousness or 'family resemblances'. We may find the preparatory state, which is expressed as craving, has a similar theme to other nondrug-related preparatory states, which may share similar feelings of inadequacy, or excitement, or desire to escape, or express a lack in the current situation. The following case examples are taken from the author's smoking research:

A female smoker craves cigarettes in certain social situations. The craving is so strong that she will interrupt the flow of social communication in order to find a cigarette. She feels she cannot continue without a smoke. Points at which craving is transformed into an urge are fairly precise. She is sitting down at a meeting when a group of friends arrive and stand in front of her. She doesn't feel the urge to smoke when she is relaxing alone. She gets up to join them with her thoughts on the conversation and she prepares to enter it. When she is in the group, she is aware of an absence in her hands, which develops into the thought that she must get a cigarette. She now asks for one.

There are several distinct preparatory phases involved here that mature and roll into one. But there is a key preparatory theme that emerges if we look across similar situations. She does not have the same craving when talking with superiors or with children, it is mostly with colleagues of the same status. In many ways talking with colleagues is for her a most vulnerable situation, since it is with peers that she has most liberty to interact and expose herself and most chance of being judged. So, when she enters an interaction like this one she is preparing to pay attention, but with the consequence that she may be judged for it and the further consequences this will have. This type of preparation involves a hesitant style of interaction, an attention to self and heightened awareness of body position and manipulations and she becomes more likely to perceive a lack or absence of something about herself. The craving 'act' in this case is embedded in the surrounding act of preparing for a stressful social interaction.

An editor cannot concentrate on writing a text without a cigarette. She sits down prepared for a difficult job, and as soon as she is in place her first act is to reach for a cigarette to light up and then to start to edit the text, taking breaks every now and then to have a puff. The preparation for a difficult task and the structuring of the performance create a tension, a rigid expectation that requires also preparing for a distraction so that the work becomes tolerable. Restructuring work expectations is a priority here in overcoming craving.

A manual worker smokes when relaxed and taking a break. He finds it difficult to do nothing. He feels doing nothing is unproductive. When the time for his break arrives he sits down preparing for something lacking in the situation. He reports feeling agitated when doing nothing and this agitation accentuates the craving for a cigarette. Ironically, smoking agitates him further, but he reports feeling better smoking and claims smoking relaxes him despite its stimulant properties.

The preparation to smoke in these cases is part of a chain of prior preparations and anticipations of which the person is often not aware. Once the smoker has set themselves up for a cigarette, whether the preparation is primarily cognitive or behavioural, all the other aspects and associations of 'craving' seem to fall in around the preparatory state. This may explain why sometimes thoughts of use, or sensations, follow on one another with no set priority. Once the state is triggered it will continue on under its own momentum.

This notion of a flow of preparatory stages is similar to, say, Marlatt and Gordon's (1985) idea of how a drinker may come to make an apparently irrelevant decision. They give the example of a drinker who plans a drive but, through a series of apparently unrelated decisions, ends up outside his favourite bar. The notion here is that the person consciously or unconsiously may set themselves up for craving.

However, the preparatory notion is more specific; it does not ascribe a wilful motivation, and relates to the immediate experience of craving. The clinical implications also differ from Marlatt and Gordon's example since the first step in a descriptive-based treatment is to shift the awareness of the person away from a temporal-based perspective on craving (that it is about cigarettes) to a detection of the earlier preparatory state and the link with other similar situation-specific feelings.

Changing the preparatory state itself can be effectively approached through a role therapy, which encompasses all the cognitive, social and physiological aspects of the state without necessarily focusing on any one in particular; just the intentional theme of the role is needed. A very different physiological response results from whether, for example, the person plays the role of victim, spectator or master of a stressful scenario. Imagery and script can be devised in collaboration with the client to support an alternative narrative. A useful strategy can be to advise the person to prepare for the role antagonistic to the preparatory craving state. So if, for example, the craving is embedded in the desire to concentrate, preparation can focus on adopting a more relaxed role to the task. The role-playing strategy involves constructing a serious and comprehensive role rehearsal around the activity, from the moment the future activity is conceived until it is actually approached. It is no use waiting until the person is already immersed in their previous role and the 'craving' has already emerged as part of the habitual preparation.

The manual labourer in the example above was able to construct a role for himself as someone who read during his break. Reading was for him antagonistic to smoking. This role change did not just involve 'behavioral substitution', but involved literally redefining his role in entering the situation. The change encompassed the flow of experience throughout the scene: what he thought about; where he looked; the way he came to sit down; how he placed the book; what he anticipated doing while he read and after he finished reading.

RE-EVALUATION OF THE MEANING OF ADDICTION

If craving is no more than a label attached to a preparatory state and is more reflective of the person than of the addiction, then a cornerstone of 'addiction' theories has disappeared. If craving does not indicate control by the drug then the drug is not 'addictive'. In the same way that 'craving' is no more than a series of qualitatively-different preparatory states, so addiction is no more than a series of qualitatively-different self-medication acts tied more to personal goals and behavioural style than to drug effects.

Indeed, studies do show that conditions of acquiring an addiction and of breaking addiction vary considerably with personal circumstances. Physicians who become dependent often do so because of unrealised goal expectations. Conversely, adolescent addiction is often a consequence of peer pressure and may resolve itself as more responsibilities are taken up in later life (Peele 1985). A general theory of gambling proposes that gambling meets the personal need to confirm existence, affirm worth and produce affects (Kusyszyn 1990). In other words, addiction is wound up with regulation of worth, esteem and interpersonal relations.

Marsh (1984) found those who quit smoking had a powerful set of beliefs in non-smoking and had lost faith in what smoking could do for them. The pattern of relapse and remission was marked by changes in social images and expectations, and relapse occurred when smoking fitted favourably into social needs rather than biological ones. Vaillant (1983) noted that the most significant prognostic factor in alcoholics was whether they had anything to lose socially by drinking. Working and marital conditions seemed mostly responsible for positive outcome in alcoholics.

Widening the context of 'addiction' to include social factors also brings out the important aspect of wider societal definitions of 'addiction'. The label 'addiction' is applied now to a wide variety of behaviours where the person is seen to attach their ego to another person or substance, for example, tele-addict, junk-food addict, dependent relationship, etc. Where the person is self-administering to needs responsibly, they are seen as self-regulating. But where the behaviour is perceived as outside of the permissible limits for the individual to act, then the person is considered 'addicted'.

Stein (1990) has explored clinical ideologies and practices towards alcoholism as cultural metaphors and he suggests that in an era of neo-puritanism, addicts serve as reservoirs of 'badness' for mainstream society. The goal of his meaning-centred anthropological discourse is to locate the phenomenon of alcoholism and other labelled 'chemical addictions' in contemporary society and to offer an ethnographic model of the cultural milieu in which it occurs.

In conclusion, craving and addiction may be best understood in a person-centred context rather than the drug-centred context usually ascribed to them. Applying a descriptive analysis provides us with a wider view of how to organise the interacting levels of cognitive factors, behaviour and physiology involving drug use without jumping too prematurely to causal models, and so leaning too heavily on received wisdom.

SUMMARY

Craving is the emotion which accompanies the behavioural repertoire of addiction, and may be both independent of and more important than withdrawal experiences in maintaining maladaptive habits. Craving can be viewed in the context of attributional theories of emotion and motivation, in that the craved object is ascribed properties which are expected to decrease an ahedonic mode of being and/or enhance well-being. There is some evidence, notably from the benzodiazepine-withdrawal literature, that personality variables predict withdrawal more than quantity of withdrawn substance. It is argued that cognitive factors in craving are more intimately involved with preparation and anticipation of current tasks than to drug-related physiological factors. It is suggested that the act of craving reflects personal coping style and can be explored qualitatively by looking for resemblances with the way the person copes in other situations, rather than assuming that craving can be explained through drug effects.

Chapter 8

Capgras syndrome and delusions of misidentification

Humans have a highly-developed visual discriminatory ability, and this is especially so when the stimuli to discriminate are human faces. Facial recognition has long been of fascination to psychologists involved in the study of visual perception and social development. The infant is able to fixate on the eyes of others days after birth and reciprocate gaze. In this sense, the child exhibits a basic mode of social behaviour very early in its life. It has been suggested that reciprocation of eye contact is an innate response to the gaze of others at this developmental stage. Though initially an infant makes social-approach gestures to virtually any human company, the child quickly discriminates between the faces of caretakers and those of strangers and becomes distressed in the presence of the latter, a response known as 'stranger anxiety'. As humans mature, the level of discrimination involved in facial recognition becomes highly sophisticated, so that an individual can retain visual information of the faces of literally hundreds of other people. Visual facial data is processed rapidly, so that recognition usually occurs without resort to lengthy consideration.

The neurologist Ian Meadows (1974) reflects that

> It should be realised that recognition of faces is a most complex and sophisticated visual achievement which is particularly gestalt-like in nature, for most faces are resistant to verbal interpretation. We can each probably recognise over 1,000 faces, many of which differ in fine rather than gross detail, but we do this in a manner which it is quite impossible to convey verbally. It depends on learning what are essentially visual pattern discriminations of great complexity.
>
> (Meadows 1974)

Retention can also be effected with speed, so that as little as a fraction of a second's exposure is required for familiarisation with a new face. It is not surprising that human beings have a highly-developed mechanism to differentiate between fellow members of the same species. Humans are gregarious creatures who tend to function in groups for their survival. Without the ability to identify members of the same group and distinguish them from members of other groups, social cohesiveness would break down. In everyday life, false recognition of familiar persons is rare, as witnessed by the embarrassment and apologetic stance of a person who has wrongly greeted a stranger, mistaking that person for a long-lost friend. Correct identification of familiar others is crucial, without which we would be unable to respond selectively to our social milieu.

THE MISIDENTIFICATION SYNDROMES

There are a variety of dysfunctional processes that are associated with breakdown of facial discriminative ability, so that misidentification takes place. The misidentification can either be positive or negative. In positive misidentification, the subject is over-inclusive, so that, for example, strangers may be greeted as relatives or friends. By contrast, in negative misidentification, familiar persons are not recognised as such. In gross brain damage, a patient may fail to recognise his or her spouse and deny any knowledge of ever having set eyes on that person before. Sometimes, previous exposure to a face has no bearing on recognition; facial characteristics cease to be cues by which individuals are identified. This presentation is one of facial agnosia, or prosopagnosia.

In prosopagnosia, the patient may be able to discriminate between and recognise persons by other means, such as their style of dress, posture or tone of voice, but in terms of visual discrimination of faces, the patient is effectively blind to features that differentiate one person from another. The ability to recognise everyday objects is well preserved in the prosopagnosic patient, and sometimes these patients use other strategies apart from facial recognition to identify specific friends and relatives, such as attending to tone of voice, style of clothing or body posture. Some patients have been known to discriminate between individuals on the basis of their spectacles, or a fine detail of facial characteristics, such as a mole or the shape of a receding hairline, but the overall shape and visual organisation of the face has no significance for recognition purposes.

There is a statistical association between organic problems of a neurological nature and person misidentification. Misidentification syndromes are positively correlated with the onset of dementia (e.g. Lipkin 1988). Crichton and Lewis (1990) have reported the occurrence of delusional misidentification in association with AIDS, where there has been evidence of neurological degeneration of the central nervous system.

CAPGRAS SYNDROME

An uncommon form of negative misidentification occurs when the patient asserts that a person well known to him or her is a double of the real person. The object of this belief almost invariably involves specific persons with whom there is a special familiarity or emotional tie. This dysfunction is known as Capgras syndrome. Christodoulou makes the following comment: 'The syndrome of Capgras is the delusional negation of the identity of a familiar person (or persons) in which the patient believes that the misidentified and the familiar persons are identical physically but different psychologically' (Christodoulou 1977: 65). Capgras syndrome differs from complete poverty of recognition in that in Capgras, the 'imposter' is correctly recognised as resembling the 'real' person. For example, Anderson (1988) described a 47-year-old man who, on meeting his brother, became convinced that he was in the company of a person who was pretending to be the brother. Capgras is therefore the delusion that a specific person, or persons, have been replaced by near-identical doubles, who are imposters. The syndrome was first described by Capgras and Reboul-Lachaux (1923). Capgras syndrome is a residual delusion which is as distinctive as it is colourful.

A variant of Capgras has been recorded in the literature, consisting of the misidentification of pets and inanimate objects. An example of the latter is a case quoted by Coleman (1933) in which a female patient suddenly developed the conviction that some personal letters in her possession, which she re-read from time to time, were fakes and not the originals. In another, more recent, example, a 59-year-old female patient developed the conviction that her cups and saucers had been replaced with replicas, together with various other household objects, such as the gas fire and a picture hanging on the wall (Abed and Fewtrell 1990). In her retrospective account of the delusion, she described feeling that the familiar objects 'seemed different'. She began searching for finer detail, such as hair-line cracks in the crockery and found some which she had not noticed before. We will refer back to the progression of subjective events described in Abed and Fewtrell's case later in this chapter. The delusion of the replacement of inanimate objects is commonly viewed as a variant of Capgras because the form of the dysfunction is the same in both, while the content of both is related in theme.

Berson (1983), in a review of 133 cases of Capgras syndrome, noted a firm diagnosis of schizophrenia in over half. Almost a quarter were diagnosed as having an organic disorder, while 13 per cent exhibited features of bi-polar affective disorder. Many case examples of Capgras syndrome reported in the literature occur in association with neurological illness, such as dementia (Lipkin 1988) and posterior pituitary tumour (Anderson 1988). Phenomenologically-minded clinicians do not challenge this fact, since the occurrence of organic brain disease in some patients exhibiting the Capgras delusion is incontrovertible. Yet the position of phenomenologists is that a delusion is a presentation of the psyche, that is, it reflects an aspect of consciousness and therefore lies within a 'sphere of influence' that is outside of the bounds of the physical. What, then, is the role of phenomenological study in such cases? How can a phenomenological approach illuminate aspects of the syndrome, when the phenomenon is itself linked in some way to a physical entity?

Jaspers made the following comments on the relationship between neurological entities and material pertaining to the psychic (psychological) sphere:

Investigation of somatic function, including the most complex cortical activity, is bound up with investigation of psychic function, and the unity of the soma and psyche seems indisputable. Yet we must remember that neither line of enquiry encounters the other so directly that we can speak of some specific psychic event as directly associated with some specific somatic event or of an actual parallelism. The situation is analagous with the exploration of an unknown continent from opposite directions, where the explorers never meet because of impenetrable country that intervenes.

(Jaspers 1963)

Jaspers adopted the view that there is an aetiological link between disorders definable on a physical basis, particularly neurological disorders, and psychological symptoms, particularly those in which there is an information-processing deficit. However, he expressed concern about the vacuum of knowledge pertaining to the transformation of neurological mechanisms to psychological processes. He continues:

We only know the end links in the chain of causation from soma to psyche and vice versa and from both these terminal points we endeavour to advance. Neurology has discovered that the cortex with the brain-stem provides the organ most closely associated with psychic function and its researches have reached their highest peak so far in the the theory of aphasia, agnosia and apraxia. It seems, however, as if the further neurology advances, the further the psyche recedes; psychopathology on the other hand explores the psyche to the limits of consciousness but finds at these limits no somatic process directly associated with such phenomena as delusional ideas, spontaneous affects and hallucinations.

(Jaspers 1963)

Jaspers appeared to view many aspects of psychological disturbance as causally linked to neuropathology, but was dissatisfied with the lack of clarity in the relationship between diseases of the central nervous system and consciousness-mediated phenomena. Jaspers observed that specific features of psychopathology cannot be predicted from a given lesion or degenerative CNS disease process.

Capgras syndrome provides an invaluable opportunity to consider advances in the neurological and psychopathological sequelae of a delusion. Neither is adequate in explaining the cognitive manifestation in question, but some of the 'impenetrable country' between the two 'spheres of influence', to use Jasper's terminology, has been eroded by empirical findings and clinical observation. It is inconceivable that the presence of a tumour or lesion, or cerebral atrophy gives rise to a delusional belief of specific content directly. The proposition is facile, since semantic structure and communicated meaning bears no direct relation with organic matter. A lesion and a delusion are quanta which are causally incompatible without the introduction of mediating processes. Therefore, to understand causal links, it is necessary to form a conceptualisation of the intervening variables which account for the transformation of the neurological entities, i.e. physical matter, into ideational phenomena, e.g. delusional belief. How, then, might some of the Jasperian 'impenetrable ground' be cleared in the context of Capgras? What role does neuropathology play in a process culminating in a delusional belief in the replacement of close others by replicas?

First, let us look at some clinical details of Capgras patients, including physical pathology known to accompany the delusion, ideational components and the affective atmosphere in which the delusion takes place.

SOME CASE EXAMPLES INVOLVING THE CAPGRAS DELUSION

Christodoulou (1977) described the clinical picture associated with the Capgras delusion in a number of patients, some of which are described below. The first was a 43-year-old woman who, at the age of 31, accused her husband of infidelity. Initially, she began acting oddly and expressed hypochondriacal ideas. After the death of her mother, she stopped speaking to her husband and later refused to speak to anyone in her village apart from her own children and domestic pets. She became progressively bizarre and unpredictable, though, to the relief of her relatives, she began speaking again, initially to her father. Her relatives assumed that she was her old self again, until she reported to the police that her husband had died and had been replaced by an identical-looking man. She wore a black dress to mourn her 'late' husband and refused to sleep with his 'double', whom she angrily ordered out of the house, demanding that he should sleep with his own wife. Later, she reported to the police that the 'double' invited other men into the house and that they had all attempted to rape her. She also claimed that her possessions had been taken away by her husband's 'imposter' and been replaced by identical-looking objects.

On admission to hospital, she was dressed in black. When asked about her marital status, she described herself as a widow. Her husband had, in fact, brought her into hospital; when asked about his identity, she replied that she did not know him, and then suddenly turned to him and hit him in the face. She was subsequently diagnosed as suffering from paranoid schizophrenia.

The second patient was a 68-year-old married woman who was prone to angry outbursts of shouting at night, much to the displeasure of her neighbours. She accused her family doctor, daughter and psychiatrist of impersonating the real people. She was deeply mistrustful and suspicious, and expressed persecutory delusions, such as that 'refridgeration gas' had been pumped into her flat and poison put in her bath. She claimed that the 'imposters' of her daughter and psychiatrist wore masks to try and deceive her, but said that she was able to detect differences in the appearance of one of the 'imposter's' teeth, which she held to be slightly different from her daughter's, while the 'stooge' psychiatrist was not as smart as the 'real' psychiatrist.

The patient presented with Parkinsonian features. Neurological tests revealed that she had an abnormal EEG. Atrophy of the frontal lobes was suggested by a CAT scan. The overall picture therefore involved considerable evidence of degenerative organic pathology.

The third patient was a 24-year-old man who was admitted to hospital from a home setting in which there had been considerable marital stress. The patient presented with the conviction that his wife had been replaced by a double. It was revealed from the history that the patient had had a skull fracture at the age of 2, with neurological sequelae, and a convulsion at the age of 11. He described a domestic picture of a distraught wife and considerable disharmony between the couple. Neurological examination and physical and psychometric testing revealed no abnormality in current signs or performance.

From the recent history it was noted that he had initially become suspicious of his superiors at work and he began to have angry outbursts at home. He started to believe that he was being pursued, and this belief had a paranoid flavour. On the ward, he became convinced that his wife was an imposter sent to visit him by unknown persecutors. Further investigation revealed that he had had this conviction several times previously, coinciding with significant life events, such as the birth of the couple's first child and during each job transfer. Sometimes, the delusion had extended to his mother and his son.

On the ward, the patient presented photographs of his wife and pointed out small details of her appearance which he claimed were evidence that the person in the photograph was the 'different' woman who visited him. Shortly afterwards, he relocated to another geographic area, a life event which, based on historical evidence, was likely to exacerbate the clinical picture. He developed the belief that voices from the radio were talking to him directly and he became acutely disturbed while on leave. He returned to hospital with persecutory delusions, which replaced the Capgras ideation.

THEORIES OF THE PATHOGENESIS OF THE CAPGRAS DELUSION

Because of the absence of a known mechanism mediating the Capgras picture and the appearance of the delusion within a variety of different clinical presentations, Enoch and Trethowan (1967) prefer to adopt the term 'Capgras symptom' rather than 'Capgras syndrome'. A syndrome is defined as a group of prominent symptoms that coexist, forming a set of characteristics which share a temporal relationship. For Enoch and Trethowan, there are insufficient coexisting features to warrant the term 'syndrome'. Enoch and Trethowan consider that the overall psychopathological state varies so much across patients that there are no particular features occurring in parsimony with the ideational component of the Capgras phenomenon with sufficient consistency across patients to form a cluster of multiple psychological symptoms. However, the term 'Capgras syndrome' has remained. Though this may be partly out of several decades of habitual use, there is also a general consensus that there is a cluster of features present, though the cluster does not involve major first-rank diagnostic criteria of the so-called 'syndrome'.

In assessing the nature of a phenomenon, it is important to have knowledge of concomitant factors that surround the thing itself, particularly the processes which are simultaneously part of the psychological field. Without taking a 'cross-section' of mental activity, it is impossible to form an impression of its *Dasein* structure. The clinical picture concomitant with Capgras ideation appears to vary from patient to patient, as the above case examples provided by Christodoulou (1977) and the literature review of Berson (1983) suggest.

It has been noted that the Capgras delusion can appear at any time of a psychosis, waxing and waning irrespective of the intensity and course of a schizophrenic episode (Enoch and Trethowan 1967). Patients in whom the Capgras delusion superimposes a wider system of delusions may therefore show fluctuation in the intensity of the major psychosis, independently of the Capgras delusion itself. At any given time, the Capgras conviction may appear or re-appear as part of the cognitive activity of a psychotic patient, but its appearance as part of the mental state cannot be predicted by the course of the overall psychopathology. Sometimes, the monosymptomatic delusion persists long after the major psychosis has resolved. Hence, the relationship between schizophrenia and Capgras is obscure, but it is clear that the Capgras delusion is not merely a schizophrenic symptom.

Neurological models of the pathogenesis of Capgras

Enoch and Trethowan (1991) point out that since 1970, around 100 Capgras cases have been reported to exhibit neurological signs, some verified by CT scan. These authors and Christodoulou (1991) therefore suggest that the Capgras delusion has an organic basis. The argument is supported by Cutting (1991), who finds a link between all the misidentification syndromes and right-hemisphere dysfunction. Lewis (1987) suggests that Capgras ideation is the product of confabulation. Confabulation is a falsification of memory which occurs in clear consciousness, but associated with amnesia following neurological disease (Berlyne 1972). Korsakov patients often confabulate, in the form of constructing fantastic stories, or by filling out gaps in memory by making up accounts of activities that the patient is unable to recall from recent memory. The problem with Lewis's hypothesis is that the Capgras patient does not conform to the clinical pattern of confabulation; the patients' accounts are highly specific and are not expansive. If amnesia of the close other occurs, the presence of confabulation fails to explain why the patient generates the delusion to provide explanation.

Recently, there has been some reconsideration of Capgras as a manifestation of prosopagnosia, i.e. an agnosia of faces (Hayman and Abrams 1977; Schraberg and Weitzel 1979; Bidault *et al.* 1986). The latter authors administered a test of facial recognition to ten subjects exhibiting misidentification of persons. Cutting (1991), though supporting the notion of an organic basis to Capgras, casts doubt on the presence of prosopagnosia based on Bidault *et al.*'s (1986) data, suggesting that the performance of Bidault *et al.*'s subjects was superior to that expected of prosopagnosic subjects. Nonetheless, Hayman and Abrams (1977) argue that the link between organic dysfunction and the dysfunction of consciousness is a breakdown in pattern recognition, and that a lesion causes a breakdown of visual discrimination. There is little evidence to support this view.

We would suggest that reception of the distal stimulus must remain unimpaired in the delusions of doubles to enable the 'imposter' or 'duplicate' to be positively identified as a double of the real person or object. In this sense, there is no element of misidentification of the physical characteristics of the distal stimulus, since patients will stress the similarity between the real people and their supposed doubles. In terms of visual discrimination, performance appears to remain perfectly normal, the 'imposter' being placed in the same lookalike category as the original person. For this reason alone, it is unlikely that Capgras can be explained in terms of the hypotheses forwarded by Hayman and Abrams (1977), i.e. that there is primary impairment involving distorted internal representation of the visual field.

Enoch (1986) reiterated the point that prosopagnosia (and, by implication, any other agnosia) is quite distinct from the phenomenon of Capgras. In the latter, the perceptual process moves from the known to the unknown object (the double), while in the positive misidentification syndromes, strangers are greeted as friends, and perception moves from the unknown to the known. Enoch also pointed out a second distinction, which is that prosopagnosia is often unstable, so that a reversal of the agnosia can occur, rendering correct identification possible again. In comparison, misidentification in Capgras patients exhibits erroneous conviction relatively more consistently over time. It is also of interest to note that, despite the profound perceptual disturbance in prosopagnosia, there is no recorded case of it being associated with delusion-formation. By contrast, Capgras is relatively stable, the misidentification becoming more permanent, and is accompanied by stable delusional activity. Furthermore, the misidentification in Capgras is limited to specific people or objects and, unlike the agnosias, is selective and not generalised.

Cutting (1991) discusses the evidence that has accumulated over recent years linking the misidentification syndromes, including Capgras delusion, to right-sided brain pathology. He quotes a case in which a male patient with extensive head injuries, involving the frontal, temporal and parietal regions, was convinced that friends, relatives and his pet cat were duplicates. As with many other Capgras patients, he showed evidence of meticulous attention to detail, so that the presence of previously unnoticed characteristics were attended to, which were then used as proof that duplication had taken place. In the instance of the pet cat, the patient noticed a scar on the pet's ear, which he had never seen before, and this newly discovered feature of the cat's appearance was taken to reinforce the delusion of replacement. Cutting's patient also developed the delusion that the hospital in which he was residing was not genuine and that he himself was not the same person, since one of his teeth was missing and a callous on his foot differed from that which he recollected as his own.

Neurological factors are obviously of questionable relevance to the minority of patients who present with the Capgras delusion alone, and to the majority of Capgras patients who present with a functional disorder. However, some of the reports citing the apparent absence of organicity are several years old, and organicity was often not thoroughly investigated and therefore cannot be ruled out. Also, the clinical picture at the time of examination is unlikely to contain a discernable neuropathology when the latter is of recent, insidious onset. Since the 1980s, an association of schizophrenia and CNS ventricular dilation has become increasingly apparent in a significant minority of schizophrenic patients, rendering the organicity hypothesis of possible relevance to Capgras cases occurring in a major 'functional' psychosis (Weinberger, 1984).

The delusion presented in the *absence* of a major functional psychosis, and in the absence of any known neurological disease process in a patient reported by Abed and Fewtrell (1990). The patient was a 55-year-old married woman who worked as a packer in a factory. There had been some changes in the workplace, in that she had recently been transferred to a different type of work, which prevented her from receiving her usual weekly bonus. She was angry about this change, which was brought about without consultation. A week later, she telephoned her workplace to say she was unwell, claiming that something strange was going on in her head. She became uncharacteristically abusive and irritable with her husband and began to withdraw. She began exhibiting bizarre behaviour, such as ripping up magazines and catalogues. She packed all her clothes into large bin-bags for disposal, claiming that the clothes were not hers and expressed the view that a number of familiar household objects were not her own and had been replaced by near-identical duplicates.

The patient was admitted to hospital, where she initially refused to eat the food, saying that it would be hypocritical to do so because there was no justification for her being there. She was prescribed oral chlorpromazine. Two weeks after admission, she became more sociable and began to express doubts about whether the household items had really changed. Shortly afterwards, she was discharged, but provided us with a retrospective account of the delusion-formation: she recalled that she began to feel 'odd' during the period in which she felt restless and angry following what she, and the majority of her work collegues, considered to be disrespectful gestures from the factory management. She was at home, doing some cleaning, when she looked up to find that her surroundings appeared strangely unfamiliar, as if she had never seen them before. She recalled thinking that everything was in its usual place but she was troubled by the impression that nothing looked quite the same, and was distressed by the novel appearance that her everyday possessions, such as ornaments and crockery, had taken on. She began looking closely at some of the items that looked different and discovered characteristics of some of them which she had not noticed before. She became convinced that hair-line cracks in her tea cups were new and that the painting of a tiger in the living room had whiskers, whereas she believed that the painting she originally bought had not. She then reached the conclusion that these items, together with the gas fire and the road sign outside her window, had been mysteriously replaced by replicas.

Capgras and Reboul-Lachaux (1923) also noted this excessive attention to detail in their own patients, and used the phrase 'agnosia due to great attention' to reflect the role of the inappropriate attentional focusing in generating the delusion of duplication. During this process, the overall appearance of the close others becomes poorly attended to as the focus of awareness shifts to irrelevant minutae, so that, in effect, the gestalt of the distal stimulus is obscured and becomes lost.

Psychoanalytic theory and the pathogenesis of Capgras

There has been considerable speculation among psychoanalysts regarding the pathogenesis of Capgras. The psychoanalytic explanation of the formation of the delusion is that the belief arises out of an unconscious wish to give the human object a different identity. Joseph Capgras himself initially put forward the hypothesis that the dysfunction was a misinterpretation of the external stimulus arising primarily from an aberrant emotional state. Capgras et al. (1924) viewed the delusion as serving the function of coping with unacceptable depersonalisation. Essentially, their hypothesis proposed that the delusion is generated to provide a rationale to justify a feeling of strangeness and unfamiliarity. Capgras and his colleagues went on to add a psychoanalytic dimension to the hypothesis. For example, Capgras and Carette (1924) proposed that the delusion was constructed to divert the incestuous thoughts of their patient for her father.

Later, psychodynamic theory considered the delusion to be generated by ambivalent feelings towards an individual of emotional significance to the patient. Idealisation of the significant other conflicts with the development of emotions of loathing and hate. In object-relations theory terms, the significant other acquires two personas in the eyes of the patient and is construed as both a good and a bad object. This becomes too much for the ego to tolerate and therefore a splitting occurs, in which the bad qualities of the close other are attributed to an imposter. Positive feelings toward the significant other are hence preserved, and negative, painful emotions attributable to the close other are denied, though the patient is then left to deal with the presence of the 'impersonator', who can be loathed with justification as a fraudulent individual of sinister character. An example of psychoanalytic formulation of the dysfunction is provided by Enoch (1986).

The psychoanalytic theory of splitting and projection runs into difficulties in explaining the misidentification of inanimate objects. It is feasible that some objects, such as those of sentimental value, will be of emotional significance to their owner and may come to symbolise aspects of a significant close other person with whom the objects have associations. Coleman (1933) provides a fitting example, of a patient who developed a delusion that her love letters had been replaced. However, it is difficult to see how some objects reportedly incorporated into the Capgras delusion have any emotional significance at all. In the case reported by Abed and Fewtrell (1990), for example, it is unlikely that there was any substantial affective investment in the road sign in the street, or the gas fire in the living room.

The second difficulty for psychoanalytic theory is the interchangeability of the individuals who become incorporated in the delusion. Some patients exhibit a regular shift in the person or persons considered to have been duplicated. Psychoanalytic prediction would require the Capgras patient to have considerable emotional investment in the object of perceived duplication, but in some case examples the delusion of duplication involves objects of no obvious emotional significance.

Phenomenological approaches to Capgras

In Chapter 1, we contrasted psychoanalytic thinking and the medical approach with that of phenomenology. Psychoanalysis is 'theory-driven' and is therefore limited to an explanation bound by the parameters of psychoanalytic theory itself. Similarly, medicine is steeped in the science of anatomy and physiology, and therefore explanatory concepts are restricted to the realm of the physical. A phenomenological analysis, on the other hand, is driven by the data of consciousness and fulfils the role of constructing a full picture of the psychic phenomena involved. Jaspers (1963) held the conviction that the key to explanation and understanding is to construct a good description of subjective events, incorporating all observable entities into an holistic framework of 'static analysis' (see Chapter 10). This approach is based on the premise that functional interrelationships between psychological events cannot be ascertained before the global experience is firmly established, to form the basis for further explanatory 'genetic' analysis. Various phenomenological analyses of the Capgras syndrome have been carried out, notably by Christodoulou (1986b) and Sims (1986). Both take the perspective that visual discrimination remains well preserved, but that the intact visual percept is ascribed new meaning.

Because Capgras occurs in the context of various diagnostic states, it is legitimate to investigate the presence of the psychic phenomena which coexist with all the diagnoses in question. Todd (1957), while observing the syndrome alongside affective disorder and schizophrenia, noted the presence of depersonalisation as a feature common to patients in both these diagnostic groups. For Todd (1957), depersonalisation phenomena are sufficient for precipitation of an altered emotional response to a stimulus which previously elicited a predictable and familiar sensation, generating the feeling of estrangement also described by Sims (1986) and Anderson (1988). Depersonalisation would fit the subjective conditions that can occur within an intellectually well-preserved subject, but in which the feeling quality of perception is altered, particularily when the 'jamais vu' variant of derealisation is present.

Anderson (1988) has attempted to link the *jamais vu* quality of perception in Capgras patients to neurological abnormality. He suggests that there is a breakdown of communication between the CNS structures handling incoming visual information and the emotional projection areas of the cortex responsible for reacting to the stimulus by means of a covert emotional response. He suggests that neurological abnormality translates into psychological feelings of unfamiliarity when the organic lesion interferes with the parts of the CNS which imbue a familiar percept with its habitual emotional significance. The single case which Anderson presented was found to have a posterior pituitary tumour, which he has suggested intruded into cortical areas implicated in emotional recognition. Anderson postulates that the patient developed the delusion in response to the perception of persons familiar to him being accompanied by a flat or unfamiliar emotional response. The hypothesis of inappropriate emotional response in the face of a familiar stimulus is a position that has gained ground in phenomenological circles.

Sims's hypothesis differentiates between two perceptual processes: first, reception of the distal stimulus, and second, the connotation this percept is given. Sims (1986), like Anderson, postulated that the intact percept is imbued with novel, inappropriate, emotional meaning, so that the feeling quality accompanying the familiar stimulus is unfamiliar. Sims has suggested that the Capgras syndrome seen in schizophrenia arises out of delusional perception. The intact percept is attributed new meaning, delusional perception comprising the sudden and spontaneous attribution of new, bizarre significance to external stimulus events, the distal features of which remain unchanged and are accurately perceived by the subject. During delusional perception, a spontaneous, inappropriate reassessment is made, which bears no relation to the meaning-matrix in which the attended percept is normally embedded. The content of thinking associated with delusional perception is said to emerge in an atmosphere of intense felt-meaning. Sims (1988: 97) feels that, around the onset of Capgras, subjects have usually had ambivalent feelings towards the person who is believed to have been replicated.

Delusional beliefs characteristically enter consciousness spontaneously as sudden, immediate cognitions. Though the content of the delusion is false, the belief is experienced as a remarkable insight, which is received with considerable relief and tension reduction. Suddenly, the patient feels that the world has become comprehensible once more. Primary delusions are usually preceded by a period in which the patient feels puzzled and bewildered by situations and external events that are commonplace in his/her way of life, and which might under normal circumstances be perceived as mundane or lacking any particular significance. This phase is known as 'delusional mood' or 'delusional atmosphere'. Delusional perceptions are, as Mellor puts it:

> usually preceded by a state of delusional atmosphere, which is an extremely unpleasant experience, characterised by uncertainty, anxiety, depression and perplexity. Familiar objects in the environment threaten but do not concede new meanings. Suddenly, within this terrifying world, one perception stands out, because it has meaning that explains the strange experiences. This is the delusion, and with it comes a remarkable improvement in the patient's level of distress. The delusional atmosphere diminishes and the familiar meanings of other objects are no longer in doubt.
>
> (Mellor 1991)

It is therefore after exposure to the above subjective conditions that delusions are said to arise. The experience of delusional atmosphere may last for several weeks or months, during which time the patient is engaged in a constant search for the meaning behind their intuitive sense of foreboding and insecurity.

The question of whether Capgras is a primary or secondary delusion is unclear. Mellor states the following about the differentiation:

> we must distinguish between two major groups of delusions. In one group, the delusions emerge understandably from disordered mental functions such as abnormal affects, or false perceptions. In the other, the delusions do not arise from underlying abnormal phenomena, but are, in Jaspers' terminology, psychologically irreducible and statically non-understandable; these are primary delusions.

(Mellor 1991:104)

It is open to question whether the delusional ideation in Capgras is unrelated to distorted perception and abnormal affects. *Jamais vu* experiences give rise to propositional statements that reflect the perceived unfamiliarity of stimulus objects which the subject knows as familiar. This paradox, in the face of a stimulus situation involving a close other, would presumably generate propositional statements such as 'Though I know X so well, X seems somehow different, as if I had never seen X before'. If this cognition is superimposed on thought premises that reflect delusional mood, such as 'There's something strange going on, I should keep on the look-out for some kind of plot', delusions of replication become understandable: the familiar other is recognised by the subject, but takes on an apparently inexplicable novel appearance, while simultaneously, the subject is hypervigilant to sinister plots of an as yet unspecified nature. The cognitive 'palette' is consistent with the formation of hypotheses along the lines that the familiar other is being impersonated by an imposter.

There has been a recent attempt to simulate aspects of the *Dasein* structure of patients exhibiting *jamais vu* and delusional mood in normal subjects. In a recent investigation, Gilman (1993) exposed normal subjects to propositional statements typical of delusional mood and *jamais vu*, recorded in their own voices. The statements representative of *jamais vu* experiences incorporated a close other. Thus, one subject was played back statements referring to her husband, John, such as 'Although he looks the same, John seems peculiarly different, though it's difficult to work out why', and 'I've seen John thousands of times, but now he seems like a different person'. These statements were alternated with the statements representative of delusional mood, such as 'There's something going on behind my back and I'm not sure what it is'. The subjects were encouraged throughout the procedure to forward imaginative hypotheses about the source of these impressions. Four out of Gilman's thirteen subjects offered the replication of the close other as an explanatory hypothesis. This was an creative line of enquiry, which casts doubt on whether the presence of self-statements corresponding to delusional mood and derealisation experiences are sufficient to generate the delusion.

The presence of depersonalisation phenomena have been noted in Cotard's syndrome as well as in Capgras. The Cotard delusion consists of the patient's conviction that s/he is dead. Wright *et al.* (1993) address the question of the role of depersonalisation in Capgras and Cotard's syndrome and ask why the beliefs generated in each instance are different. In Capgras, depersonalisation is superimposed with paranoid affect; while in Cotard's, depression is the predominant superimposing experiential phenomenon. Wright *et al.* point out that depressive and paranoid states have opposing attributional styles. In recent work on the attributional style of depressed and paranoid patients it has been established that, whereas patients with persecutory delusions attribute unpleasant events to outside influences, depressed patients tend to attribute such changes to self (Kaney and Bentall 1989; see Chapter 10).

Therefore, Wright *et al.* (1993) view Capgras and Cotard's delusions as interactions between depersonalisation phenomena and paranoia, and depersonalisation phenomena and depression respectively. As their hypothesis goes, while the depersonalised depressive, faced with familiar persons or objects might think, for example, 'X is unreal and unfamiliar, I must have changed . . . I am dead', the depersonalised paranoid patient might think 'X is unreal and unfamiliar, X must have been replaced'. Wright *et al.* are suggesting that the propositional self-statements (of self-mortification and of duplication) are hypotheses generated by the patient to make sense of feelings of emotional estrangement, which become integrated into a rationale of either non-existence of self, or non-appearance of familiar other, depending on the direction of attribution.

The explanation of Capgras delusion-formation is incomplete, and requires a level of explanation that ties up the contradictory data concerning neuropathology. Since the majority of cases exhibit a schizophrenic disorder, and a sizeable minority have neurological lesions or a degenerative CNS disorder, a mechanism is required that can be invoked by neuropathology or functional processes. Recently, there have been some theoretical developments which go a considerable way to find a common denominator of neuropathology and schizophrenic features. Both Anderson (1988) and Ellis and Young (1990) have proposed that the Capgras delusion occurs when there is an absence of the habitual emotional response to a familiar stimulus, and suggest that, in subjects with neuropathology, damage has occurred within the neuro-anatomical pathways which imbue familiar stimuli with the affective colouration. The psychological effect of the neuropathology in Capgras therefore renders the familiar stimulus devoid of emotional connotation. Delusional perception, which is characteristic of schizophrenia, also has the effect of uncoupling a familiar stimulus from its usual emotional meaning.

SUMMARY

The phenomenological perspective forces us to examine the psychic phenomena accompanying Capgras, rather than become deflected by diagnostic concepts. This abstracts us from biological and medical 'explanations' and prompts us to consider the experiential structure surrounding the delusional ideation. Epidemiological data reveal that Capgras is rare, occurring occasionally in the context of several morbid processes, including schizophrenia and neuropathology such as brain lesions and Alzheimer's disease. The most frequent site of discrete neuropathology is in right-sided cortical lesions. The Capgras delusion provides a good opportunity to demonstrate the position of structural phenomenology with regard to a neurological problem. The issue of how the felt-meaning of the delusion arises has been a matter of intense recent debate.

It is arguable whether the content of the delusion is un-understandable. The presence of depersonalisation phenomena may invest a percept of the close other with specific propositional statements regarding inauthenticity. One of the most important issues in the genesis of Capgras-style propositional statements is how the 'as if' qualifying prefix in unreality experiences typical of depersonalisation is dropped, so that the sensory impression of unfamiliarity is taken as fact. It is suggested that the content of thinking is disordered in a manner that indicates that the Capgras patient has constructed erroneous conclusions in making sense of feelings of unreality. The (external) attributional style that paranoid subjects exhibit in the face of negative events (see Chapter 10) may go some way to providing this link. When all is said and done, depersonalisation is intrinsically unpleasant and therefore conceivably gives rise to, or comprises such a negative event.

The tendency for deluded subjects to form spontaneous, false hypotheses, through jumping to premature conclusions, and the presence of distorted attributional styles associated with specific features of psychopathology are discussed further in Chapter 10.

Chapter 9

Positive experience and states of enlightenment

THE IDEA OF OPTIMAL SUBJECTIVE STATES

Therapy is a means to an end. Generally, a therapeutic situation involves interaction between the therapist, as a provider of conditions aimed at promoting beneficial change, and the recipient, the patient or client. There is a substantial amount of literature that reviews the range of dysphoric experiences of which clients complain, maladaptive behaviours which clients exhibit, and the pathogenic milieu or events to which clients are exposed. This is the starting point, or baseline from which therapy begins. In psychiatry, there is an elaborate technological system of diagnostic categories that delineate maladaptive and dysfunctional syndromes. But what of the positive modes of being, associated with contentment, success and enlightenment? In this chapter, we are not so much concerned with psychologically-healthy life styles in their totality as much as some of the feelings and emotions which occur alongside them, particularly the quality of experience that is associated with well-being. There is a paucity of literature referring to the nature of healthy, positive experience and life style, even though one of the functions of therapy is to foster quality of life. In the literature on 'basic' emotions, positive experiences are subsumed under the concept of 'happiness' (for example, Weiner and Graham 1984; Oatley and Johnson-Laird 1987), or the concept of 'joy' (for example, Ekman 1982; Frijda 1987; Gray 1982; Izard 1972; Plutchick 1980). Though these positive feelings are integrated into a theoretical framework, the structure and information-processing ramifications of negative affect have generally been of more interest than the quality of positive experiences.

Not all states which have a positively hedonic tone are associated with well-being. Elation, euphoria and excitement are often mentioned in the context of positive hedonic tone, though the relationship between these states and well-being is tenuous; the expansive gestures that occur in hypomania are embedded in an affect of euphoria, but the behaviour typical of the hypomanic patient is often truculent and socially disruptive, and the numerous grandiose schemes of the hypomanic tend to be fantastic and unrealistic. It goes without saying that it is meaningless to talk of all hedonistic pleasure as wholesome and something to be sought after. Assessment of affect is contextual and inevitably judgemental. For example, the pleasure of the sadistic psychopath while torturing a helpless victim may be equal in intensity to that of a musician in full flow during a performance.

Optimal psychological states have been variously defined, with differing degrees of anchoring to ecological factors. Guntrip (1968) talks of the concept of 'mature dependence', and this state of affairs refers to an optimisation of transference between adults who have a symbiotic relationship in the psychodynamic sense. In mature dependence, each partner has split off from parents and has formed an ego-identity which functions autonomously, without the need for regressive dependence on guardian figures; the mature adult has resolved conflicting emotions and repressed those which are maladaptive, to the extent that he or she relates to the world in a functionally-competent fashion. Lover has replaced parent and libidinal urges have been transferred to this new love object. Regressive urges of both partners may be acted out and supported within the relationship, but, importantly, when this occurs one partner parents the other and the roles are reversible and flexible. The object-relations theory concept of mature dependence therefore expresses a way of relating with and coping with the world that has as its reference point the mode of being, which is balanced between need for nurturance and need to provide love, and the internal dynamics of the individual is healthy as long as an equilibrium is maintained between these two modes.

The concept of mature dependence is an important one, since it provides the object-relations therapist with an outline, albeit couched within theory-driven terms, of an ideal. It is a therapeutic ideal which influences the goals of treatment and gives a sense of direction to object-relations therapy, suggesting a conceptual path along which the patient is guided to get from an undesirable to a desirable point in existence. The goal is not a singular emotional experience, but a mode of operating, a means of relating in the context of an emotional relationship, and is taken as the ideal goal, which is as much ecological as it is psychodynamic. The primary ecological setting, intrinsic to the psychodynamic therapies, is the familial environment, and from within this environment, the patient progresses psychodynamically from child or regressed adult to a stage of maturity, the definition of which is couched in terms of resolution of conflict, but the evidence for which is partly overt behavioural adjustment.

Behavioural psychology has inevitably played some part in inhibiting enquiry into the feeling quality of positive states. This is because both pleasant and unpleasant experiences have been construed in the context of conditioned responses, or as reinforcers. In counter-conditioning (Wolpe 1969), the most important property of a newly-conditioned response is its ability to reciprocally inhibit a maladaptive response, rather than its subjective quality. In the context of reinforcement, positive experiences and their feeling quality have been sidestepped in favour of the stimuli that elicit them, and it is the overt effect of a *stimulus* rather than the mediating emotion or feeling state that defines a reinforcing event, and the resulting response that defines positive or negative status of the reinforcement.

The influence of behavioural doctrine is implicit in many therapeutic approaches and has helped to clarify both the aims of therapy and the means of attaining those ends. A good example is the area of assertiveness training, which is sometimes adopted as a methodological approach by therapeutic movements that do not identify strongly with the mechanistic principles of reinforcement which classical behaviourism upholds. The feministic therapies regard assertiveness as a fundamental goal, which is congruent with the philosophy of raising the decision-making power and degree of control which many women undergoing psychotherapy are lacking.

Over the past two or three decades, the concept of 'assertiveness' has become extremely fashionable in therapeutic circles. During assertiveness training, the patient is encouraged to change mode, from adopting the stance of the passive victim or the submissive subject who accepts his or her lot. The polar opposite of assertiveness is submissiveness, a way of being which is assumed to be detrimental, since the patient, in the act of submission, allows whatever conditions and demands are imposed by others to be implemented without negotiation or discussion. It is easy to understand the reasoning behind assertiveness training as a means of intervention. For example, adult female survivors of sexual abuse often find themselves trapped within a relationship with a member of the opposite sex which is unfulfilling. One of the reasons for this is that the sexually-abused subject adopts a position in the relationship which replicates the power politics of the earlier abuse. An important aspect of 'feminist therapies' is to discourage passivity and develop an orientation to personal needs that is based on equality of status between one person and another.

Assertiveness is sometimes viewed as a disposition that can replace anger, whether the angry emotion is expressed as aggression or internalised. Phelps and Austin (1987) emphasise the importance of acknowledging angry feelings rather than denying them, and advise their readers to

> identify the source of the anger. Where is it coming from? . . . Many women have lived through years of unexpressed anger. It seems a woman in this position must, when she first becomes aware of her anger, go through an angry phase, in which she is angry a great deal of the time . . . until she begins to deal with her anger appropriately and realistically. This last step is called assertive use of anger.
>
> (Phelps and Austin 1987)

Lindenfield (1992) views assertiveness as a significant development in the transformation of the role of women in society from a position of subordination to a position of greater equality. She reflects to her predominantly female readership that

> with the arrival of Women's Liberation and feminism and an awakening of a sense of power, we began to use aggressive behaviour which we perceived as powerful. Many of us simply did not realize that there was a third alternative until Assertiveness Training began to open our eyes in the 1970s. The strategies

and techniques that we learned then showed us how our needs and wants could be communicated while still respecting other people's basic human rights.

(Lindenfield 1992)

Since the majority of us are engaged for almost half our conscious lives in work-related activity, it is not surprising that occupational activity has been examined as a source of well-being. Weaver (1980) integrated the results of fifteen American surveys of work satisfaction and found an average of 88 per cent of employed people get some enjoyment from their work. In the UK, Warr (1982) found that a sizeable majority of people considered that they would continue to work if a situation arose in which it became financially unnecessary to do so. It seems, then, that employees do not necessarily work only for financial gain. In fact, there is found to be only a small correlation between job satisfaction and satisfaction with salary. This is in part explained by the finding that job satisfaction does not necessarily stem from the nature of the work itself, since employment also provides the opportunity to socialise, derive a sense of purpose and identity, and a milieu in which there is provision of structured time (Veroff *et al.* 1981). For the majority of individuals, reduction in well-being is strongly correlated with unemployment (Warr 1983).

The emphasis that behaviourists place on reward from an external source in maintaining a response repertoire ignores the human characteristic to strive for achievements in the absence of any apparent extrinsic rewards. Yet, in the absence of any external reinforcement, many human beings frequently apply themselves to a specific task for no apparent gain. For example, Csikszentmihalyi (1975) observed the working patterns of artists over several months and noted that they typically worked for sustained and prolonged periods. During this time, they demonstrated a tendency to exercise impressive powers of concentration, becoming absorbed in the act of creativity, oblivious to their surroundings. On completion of the work, many of the subjects lost interest in the product of their labours, placing it to one side or storing it, with indifference to its material value or its fate. Many people, of all walks of life and all ages, demonstrate a similar capacity for sustained attention in creative acts, in which there is no apparent gain or extrinsic reward. The play behaviour of children may be included in this category. Spiritual pursuits are described as uplifting and inspirational by many religious-minded people. These activities are in some way intrinsically rewarding, and goals in themselves. The motivational source lies as much in the process as the end product. How, then, can such motivational states be decribed and explained?

Maslow (1968) outlined the concept of self-actualisation as the discovery of one's potential and limitations. There are conflicts arising out of a discrepancy between actual capabilities and those required to achieve realisation of the ideal self. In self-actualisation, there is a coming to terms with this discrepancy and the resolution of conflicting aspirations. The feeling of self-acceptance and esteem arises out of the development of an accurate self-image, particularly a realistic assessment of actual capabilities and limitations. The conditions for self-actualisation come into play when there is an optimal balance between challenges the individual seeks and the degree of success that is derived from successful outcome of the goal-directed pursuit. To some extent, Maslow's self-actualisation concept is set in ecological terms, since self-actualisation is attained when the appropriate niche is found that provides this balance. The person feels fulfilled and contented and this is associated with a sense of personal growth and, importantly, a strong sense of identity and personal integration.

Maslow (1968) regarded human motivation as containing an intrinsic desire for progression and self-development, by transcending the ambiguities and mundanities of everyday life. Problem-solving and creativity are for Maslow natural tendencies, supplying in-built needs to realise control and abstraction from mechanistic habits, leading to what he termed 'peak experience'. This peak or optimal experience is, in Maslow's terms, a feeling state in which there is intense engagement in existence, a sense of challenge and potency. During this process there occurs what Maslow (1968) described as the 'autotelic' phenomenon, in which there is a merging of action and awareness, as if both the actor and the action were at one with each other. During the autotelic mode, he postulates the occurrence of 'loss of ego', the meaning of which corresponds to a diminution of self-conscious awareness, which capitulates to sharply focused attention on the activity itself; the subject functions spontaneously and in integrated fashion, becoming totally involved in the act, with the result that self-consciousness of the doing is minimised and the experience itself, of self interacting with environment, occupies the focus of attention. The product of these peak experiences is the feeling of a profound sense of value and satisfaction. This satisfaction arises not from extrinsic reward, but from the feeling of mastery over the life-situation that has been confronted.

The concept of peak experience was well received within humanistic psychology, not least because the thesis presented man as a being of considerable refinement and elegance, when compared with the hedonistic machine depicted by behaviourists, bent on tension reduction and gratification, or the psychoanalyst's construction of man as motivated by an essentially pathological dynamic state. The motivational source for Maslow was the feeling of achievement, the satisfaction of knowing or of creativity, rather than some external reward or tension-reduction. Central to Maslow's concept of peak experience is the successful search for meaningfulness. The idea struck a chord with psychologists of the decade, not least because of the influential work of Hebb (1955). Unlike many experimental psychologists of the era, Hebb postulated that higher organisms are not motivated exclusively by arousal reduction, but seek an optimal level of arousal. In a state of arousal deficit, the organism constructs ways of raising arousal by seeking stimulation. This idea was supported by several empirical studies, including that of Harlow (1953), who found that monkeys would work actively to seek stimulation, despite the 'biological' drives being satisfied. Harlow concluded that there was a further, psychologically-oriented motivational state, which he termed the 'curiosity drive'. Curiosity was regarded as a manifestation of the desire for understanding.

Maslow's thesis, as a theory of motivation, was said to have some shortcomings.

First, it was unclear from Maslow's account how self-actualisation could be operationally defined and achieved. Further, it was unclear from Maslow's account whether a peak experience derived from one type of activity was identical in feeling quality to a peak experience derived from another. Csikszentmihalyi (1974, 1975) began to enquire into the characteristics of the process of altruistic achievement and concluded that human beings portray the capacity to experience intense pleasure from experimentation and exploratory activities, so that the development of novel ideas and new means of expression are of major importance to motivation. He postulated that a subjective state arises in the context of such activity that was positively hedonic, instilling a sense of mastery and goal-attainment, influencing self-esteem and self-worth in a favourable direction, something that he saw as directly comparable to Maslow's concept of peak experience.

There are, of course, competing models which attempt to explain sustained goal-directed activity in the absence of extrinsic reward. Skinnerian psychologists had observed the behaviour of animals placed on a randomised contingency of reward, in which a specific response resulted in reward only occasionally; when the rewards were subsequently withdrawn completely, the partially reinforced response tends to reoccur and is resistant to extinction (see Ferster and Skinner 1957). It could therefore be argued that extrinsic reward is not necessary most of the time to maintain a behaviour and that the extrinsic reinforcement occurred outside the periods of observation. Classical conditioning theorists had also established that if an apparently neutral event was paired with a rewarding stimulus, the former would acquire some of the pleasant characteristics of the latter, by association. It was therefore possible to argue that the product of the artists' labours had secondary reinforcement status, sufficient to maintain creative behaviour. Neither of these two explanations quite fitted the data.

First, Getzels and Csikszentmihalyi (1976) concluded from their observations that those artist subjects who sought or received intrinsic reward for their labours tended to move on to other professions. With regard to children in play, extrinsic rewards can interfere with rather than increase the subsequent duration and frequency of play behaviour (Lepper and Greene 1978). Similar findings have been presented by Deci and Ryan (1985), who review a diversity of empirical data which point to the fact that when subjects are reinforced with money for engaging in the very activities they spontaneously choose and enjoy, interest and involvement in them wanes. One theoretical explanation lies in the hypothesised nature of peak experiences, which are said to be self-induced and under the autonomous control of the actor. When external contingencies of reinforcement are grafted onto this process, the feeling of autonomy and self-determination is lost, denying the actor an essential ingredient of creativity. Second, there was little or no secondary reinforcement status attached to the created art object in Csikszentmihalyi's study, since many artists simply disregarded their work on completion. It was evident that the pleasure was derived from the creative behaviour rather than the end product. Third, it is difficult for behaviouristic psychology to explain the inspiration that artists feel, sometimes expressed as a feeling of elation and 'at-oneness' with the world.

The psychoanalysts also attempted to explain artistic achievement. Freud (1957) himself explained the motivation behind creativity in terms of sublimation. In the process of sublimation, biological drives unacceptable to the ego are diverted to an energy that was said to symbolise sexual gratification. Therefore, the satisfaction of creative activity was seen as a substitute for libidinal drives. This explanation does not fit comfortably with everyday life observation, not least because degree of sexual repression is not proportional to the strength of and commitment to creative urges, and creative people are not particularly characterised by sexual repression, but rather, if anything, the opposite. Csikszentmihalyi and Csikszentmihalyi (1988) appear to accept the premise that creativity is in part inspired by the unconscious motive of resolving oedipal desire, but feel that creative expression takes on its own meaning to the artist, beyond oedipal conflict; the activity becomes 'autonomous' as a reward, becoming compartmentalised from its dynamic origins.

Csikszentmihalyi and Csikszentmihalyi (1988) have pursued the notion of the pleasure of intense engagement in constructive activity and have gone to some length to reflect upon the experiential quality of this phenomenon. Dissatisfied with Maslow's concept of peak experience, because of its ambiguity, they have attempted to elaborate upon the psychological sequelae of self-actualising events. Drawing from a diversity of studies investigating feelings associated with intense, intrinsically-rewarding effort, they conclude that there is a core process involved. These authors have adopted the view that, central to all types of activity leading to the realisation of one's potential, there are a number of characteristic experiential features which cut across the boundaries of the specific activity involved, whether it be, for example, composing music, rock climbing, painting, farming or motherhood. These authors have reviewed the results of interviews and observations, some of which have been carried out by themselves. They observe that:

> Artists, athletes, composers, dancers, scientists, and people from all walks of life, when they describe how it feels when they are doing something that is worth doing for its own sake, use terms that are interchangeable in their minutest details. This unanimity suggests that order in consciousness produces a very specific experiential state, so desirable that one wishes to replicate it as soon as possible. To this state we have given the name 'flow', using a term that many respondents used in their interviews to explain what the optimal experience felt like.
>
> (Csikszentmihalyi and Csikszentmihalyi 1988: 29)

They go on to elaborate the concept of flow experiences as an ecological state in which the subject pitches his or her abilities and resources against the challenge at hand. A flow experience occurs when there is an equilibrium between personal resourcefulness and task demand, resulting in feelings of competency when the challenge stretches capability but leads to mastery:

The universal precondition for flow is that a person should perceive that there is something for him or her to do, and that he or she is capable of doing it. In other words, optimal experience requires a balance between the challenges perceived in a given situation and the skills a person brings to it.

(1988)

In fairness to Skinnerian psychologists, the principle of shaping specifically addresses the issue of keeping task demand within the capabilities of the subject by gradually expanding the criteria for reward. In shaping, contingencies of reinforcement are arranged in such a way that the chances of success are optimised. The criteria of reward are arranged so that the required responses to be rewarded are within the scope of the subject and are subsequently increased as the subject's repertoire is developed. Therefore, the clinical application of shaping simulates those conditions considered to enhance flow. A major difference between flow and shaped behaviour is the source of reinforcement; the former being internal, the latter being extrinsic. The development of teaching machines is based on shaping and the assurance of optimal reward frequency. Over the past few years, computer games have been marketed for children and adolescents and as many parents will testify, the degree to which the young become engaged in interaction with computors is remarkable. Human–computer interaction, when viewed from the perspective of 'flow', may explain the degree of sustained absorption and concentration that otherwise distractable children exhibit.

As mastery of a given situation is realised, the challenge recedes and, as the theory goes, the subject's abilities become level with or overtake that required to meet the complexity of the task demand. At this point, boredom begins to enter the affective state and the flow experience is no longer evident. The authors view flow as of immense evolutionary significance as a motivational state which prompts the human race to constantly develop its ingenuity:

To remain in flow, one must increase the complexity of the activity by developing new skills and taking on new challenges. . . . This inner dynamic of the optimal experience is what drives the self to higher and higher levels of complexity. It is because of this spiralling complexity that people describe flow as a process of 'discovering something new'. . . . Flow forces people to stretch themselves, to always take on another challenge, to improve on their abilities.

(Csikszentmihalyi and Csikszentmihalyi 1988)

An important tenent of flow theory is the particular mental state that accompanies flow activity. Experientially, flow involves an absence of self-consciousness and the suspension of more mundane concerns, so that reaching the objective becomes the exclusive domain of consciousness. This shift in cognitive style is viewed as enhancing the powers of the intellect by the convergence of problem-solving onto the task in hand. This potentiation of perception, by the narrowing of attention (a process often referred to as 'fascination' or 'absorption' in everyday language) is considered in the light of its evolutionary significance. The acquisition of the flow state is seen as the 'buzz' that maintains a high level of exploratory output, distinguishing the human species from other animals and resulting in its mastery (or powers of destruction) over our planet. This 'buzz' is described as a feeling of harmony accompanied by a loss of self-awareness, since the activity which the self directs fills the psychological field:

> Because flow produces harmony in the self, attention can be invested totally in the activity at hand. This produces that 'merging of activity and awareness' so typical of enjoyable activities. One simply does not have enough attention left to think about anything else. A consequence of this state of affairs is that the usual preoccupations of everyday life no longer intrude to cause psychic entropy of consciousness ... the 'me' disappears in flow and the 'I' takes over.
>
> (Csikszentmihalyi and Csikszentmihalyi 1988: 33)

An interesting aspect of flow theory is its reflections on self-awareness. The authors postulate that self-awareness is often aversive. The way in which self-awareness is defined in this context corresponds closely to Jaspers's concept of excessive awareness of activity, that is, the intrusion of self-conscious attention which focuses on the experience of mental activity, rather than the mental activity itself. Experience should be taken for granted, not monitored by its beholder as it occurs:

> when the conscious is conscious of itself, not only does it become less efficient, but the experience is usually painful. . . . In flow the self is fully functioning, but not aware of itself doing it, and it can use all the attention for the task at hand. At the most challenging levels, people actually report experiencing a transcendence of self, caused by the unusually high involvement with a system of action so much more complex than what one usually encounters in everyday life. The climber feels at one with the mountain, the clouds, the rays of the sun, and the tiny bugs moving in and out of the shadow of the fingers holding to the rock. . . . When all these elements are present, consciousness is in harmony, and the self – invisible during the flow episode – emerges strengthened. The negentropic quality of the flow experience makes it autotelic, or intrinsically rewarding.
>
> (Csikszentmihalyi and Csikszentmihalyi 1988: 33)

The Csikszentmihalyis' theory is an attempt to explain the human characteristic of endeavour as the natural tendency to self-impose a task demand that is repeatedly at the limits of current capability. Given the right conditions, human beings are said to position themselves in relation to environmental demands in such a way that problem-solving and sensori-motor performance are stretched progressively. This gravitation towards challenge is construed as having immense survival value for the species. It is suggested that the human species is pre-programmed via evolved mechanisms to maintain this state of industriousness. In order to ensure the furtherance of human potential, the development of capacity and extension of resourcefulness must be intrinsically gratifying. The source of gratification is proposed as the flow experience. The optimal problem-solving state is proposed to involve a restriction of attention to the task embarked upon, a state in which consciousness of self as participator is diminished, creating channel-space for new data and hypotheses, fostering the development of novel task-oriented abstraction. It is proposed that loss of the awareness of self serves to sharpen awareness of task demand. For this to happen, there is a temporary severing of awareness of internal cues which normally distract the participant toward the biological drives and, for this to occur, diminution of self-awareness must be pre-programmed as positively hedonic when attention is focused. A mainstay of evidence in support of positively-hedonic diminution of self during periods of intense concentration is the description of deep satisfaction accompanied by a sensation often described as transcendence.

Csikszentmihalyi further proposes that the pursuit of spiritual and meditative experiences serve to enhance flow experiences, and that this is carried out by two overlapping processes. First, certain meditative states limit self-awareness and attempt to gain control over consciousness by limiting awareness to highly-specific goals. Second, the capacity to experience flow can be enhanced by the achievement of an affective state that is indifferent to somatic data: the narrowing of interoceptive receptivity results in the heightening of receptivity of other, non-biological, data of consciousness.

The notion of ideal states, and the intense feeling of satisfaction is clearly not the exclusive domain of the psychology literature. It has also been written about by theologists, particularly in relation to the concept of 'divine experience', or 'religious experience' by Christian philosophers. Of great importance to the Buddhist faith is the concept of 'nirvana', a state of being that is the cornerstone of devout religious practice.

Johansson (1969) discusses the properties and characteristics of nirvana (termed *'nibbana'* in the classical language of the Tibetan monks). *Nibbana* is a slightly altered state of consciousness, brought about by the disciplined acquisition of emotional detachment from the external world and from interoceptive feelings. Within this state, the subject becomes removed from volitional pursuit, acquiring a state of authenticity by detachment from drive reduction, since tension and conflict are ameliorated. Johansson describes nirvana as:

> a state of fulfilment in which all needs and emotions have gone, a state of calm contentment and of complete intellectual insight. It is a state of internal freedom, where all dependance, insecurity and defence have disappeared. Ethical behaviour has become second nature, and the attitude towards others is friendliness, acceptance and humility.
>
> This transformation is most often referred to as the destruction of the obsessions: sensuality, becoming, speculative views and ignorance. This is described as the end of the development, and nothing more is required.
>
> (Johansson 1969: 131)

In Western culture, particularly that of the United States, assertiveness has become associated with success, both in commerce and in personal relationships. Assertiveness is a social phenomenon, in that if one individual is more assertive relative to another, the position of the other becomes one of submission – not everyone can be assertive in society, since assertiveness implies a position of dominance, newly acquired or not, over the other person(s) in a given interaction. Within the therapies, there is a modulating principle, though generally unspoken, that assertiveness as a therapeutic target should avoid egocentricity and selfish acquisition of egocentric goals. This tentative balance becomes more tenuous when there is the prospect of commercial gain, particularly when assertiveness training is an intervention used to enhance the performance of the unassertive salesman. Ethical objectives in the commercial context are obviously more difficult to reach, since the trainer can never be fully aware of how assertive behaviour influences the repertoire of the client in the context of commercial or political gain.

Though we referred earlier to assertiveness as a disposition, its core meaning reflects behaviour rather than emotion or feeling. Nonetheless, it is clear from clinical observation that assertive behaviour has ramifications on affect and often precipitates a fundamental emotional change in the subject. Johansson (1969) considers the issue of mental-health interventions in Western society and reflects upon the often unclear philosophy that underlies them. Clearly, it is not an issue which is resolvable within the current text, but, nonetheless, it is an important subject to raise, which will doubtless receive much attention from future generations of therapists. Johansson believes that the emphasis that Buddhism gives to feeling states rather than behaviour avoids many of the social complexities that Western-style therapies generate, particularly in introducing regulation of ethical behaviour. He writes:

> The modern concept of mental health builds on a narrow balance between opposites: self-assertion and altruism, dominance and humility, strong needs and self-control, success and modesty. Both are considered important but both can be developed only to a point of equilibrium which easily leads to conflict: the ideal of harmonious integration is therefore difficult to realize.
>
> In a word, although we have found great similarities between nibbana and the concept of mental health, the differences predominate, because they are expressions of very different philosophies. The psychologist stresses society, the personal success and effectiveness in this world, the unceasing activity (towards badly defined, even dubious and contradictory, goals). The Buddha stressed the individual development to internal freedom and intelligent judgment, 'disinterested' action, balance and stability.
>
> (Johansson 1969: 136–137)

Transcendence from the mundane ways of perceiving are valued in Buddhist faith. For the Buddhist, heightened awareness comes by moving beyond verbally-encoded categorisation of things. The highest form of awareness is hence non-linguistic and devoid of propositional reflective thought. Quinney notes that

> In awareness we develop insight into the nature of concepts we use to interpret

what we are thinking in reality. We discover our attachment to concepts; and we then are able to move beyond the concepts to see the ways things are in their moment of occurrence.

(Quinney 1988: 107)

AESTHETIC EXPERIENCE

Art philosophers make a distinction between types of peak experience which stem from the act of creativity and those which are founded on the process of art appreciation. The latter is said to involve a combination of fascination and intense pleasure in the art product and is known as 'aesthetic experience', a sophisticated concept which has been the subject of much debate in art circles over the years. Philosophers of art have struggled through the ages to define the phenomenological properties of art appreciation. Aesthetic experience is the core concept which serves to delineate the quality of subjective sensation which accompanies the true appreciation of an art object.

Kant (1952) adopted the concept of 'disinterest' as a focal aspect of aesthetic pleasure, and the notion has been influential in shaping subsequent thinking. 'Disinterest' in the Kantian sense has often been misinterpreted; for Kant, to be disinterested is not the same as to be uninterested. Kant used the term 'disinterest' to outline the process whereby attention becomes directed toward the aesthetic object for its own sake, with a disposition of total unpreparedness for action; the aesthetic object has no utility value but, instead, is appreciated in its own right. Therefore, in Kant's terms, disinterest refers to an indifference to intentionality; the aesthetic-appreciative mode comprises a contemplative state of personally-disengaged interest, in which there is nothing to do except experience the object of beauty.

Bullough (1912) took a similar position when he coined the term 'psychical distance'. Bullough was one of the first psychologists to be impressed by the characteristics of aesthetic sensation. He was particularly fascinated by the subjective impression of remoteness at times of peak appreciation, and he concluded that this remoteness is an integral part of appreciation itself. He described conscious processes as turning outwards to the art form, this 'externalisation' of the direction of experience producing an abandonment of the sense of self, enabling the aesthetic content to take precedence. A similar view has been taken up by many modern writers. For example, Pole wrote:

It is natural to recall the notion of the aesthetic attitude as involving a peculiar detachment, a disengagement from the practical. To say we are detached is to say that we do not respond to the situation before us, and do not feel the need to respond, with practical actions; but such responses being excluded, whether by effort of abstraction or the knowledge that they would be out of place, we can, as we could not before, dwell in the experience.

(Pole 1983)

In aesthetic experience, the individual becomes truly 'lost in art'. The distancing is therefore not a partial retreat from the external form, but a detachment from action and all that intentionality involves, including volitional states. This leads to a subjective state in which experience of self is relegated to a secondary status, enabling the aesthetic stimulus to make a more vivid impression. The dislocation of the normal stream of conscious activity and its replacement by a unique fascination for the object of interest is an essential aspect of aesthetic experience.

Roger Fry (1937) illustrates the art appreciator's required state of abstraction from day-to-day intercourse by using the analogy of viewing a street scene from a reflection in a shop window, an effect with which we are all familiar. In real terms, the reflection closely resembles the street itself; but the reflection is separate from the real situation, and this separation has a distinctive effect on the onlooker. The street suddenly takes on a more vivid and enriched appearance. The onlooker does not feel part of the scene, and the obligation to respond to the environment, to interact with it, has gone. The reflection has removed the onlooker from the immediate circumstances. In Fry's words:

> in the mirror, it is easier to abstract ourselves completely, and look upon the changing scene as a whole. It then, at once, takes on the visionary quality, and we become true spectators, not selecting what we will see, but seeing everything equally, and thereby we come to notice a number of appearances and relations of appearances, which would have escaped our notice before, owing to that perceptual economising by selection of the impressions we will assimilate, which in life we perform by unconscious processes. The frame of the mirror, then, does to some extent turn the reflected scene from one that belongs to our actual life into one that belongs rather to the imaginative life. The frame of the mirror makes its surface into a very rudimentary work of art, since it helps us to attain to the artistic vision.
>
> (Fry 1937)

Interestingly, Fry's example is reminiscent of the perceptual experience of '*jamais vu*', a concept in psychopathology that refers to the experience of seeing even familiar objects in a totally different perspective, so that the world takes on a remarkably novel appearance despite the knowledge that nothing has actually been changed.

It is clear that the aestheticians see emotion in art as cerebral rather than somatic. Pole (1983) gives the example of an audience watching a tight-rope act. The appeal of the tight-rope is the sense of thrill and fear, arising out of anticipation that the performer may fall. This for Pole could never be a source of aesthetic pleasure, but instead would come under the category of melodrama.

> The pleasures of melodrama and the like are similar to sensational pleasures. The object functions primarily as a stimulus of a certain feeling, namely fear. The appeal of the tight-rope or the lion-tamer is the same in kind. People like to

be frightened, so long as there is no real danger, at least to themselves. I do not deny that it is always pleasing to see a feat of great precision and skill finely done; but who would go to see tight-rope walking at a foot and a half from the ground? The skill is the same.

(Pole 1983)

No doubt, for Pole, doing exactly that – i.e. lowering the tight-rope to the ground level – would be the acid test for discriminating between the sensationalists and those in the audience who were judging the performance through an aesthetic eye. Doubtless, the latter group would comprise the only people remaining seated once there was no danger to the performer!

The notion of 'emotionlessness' in art is a position that carries its own problems in incorporating the various qualities of experience purporting to be 'artistic'. Pole illuminates the problem in citing theatre as a specific theoretical difficulty, and concludes that there are grounds for excluding this medium from the aesthetic stable:

any competent dramatist must know how to work on the feelings of his audience; how to vary the tension with relief, to hint at fears, to lull them and to let them loose. The cauldron scene in *Macbeth* is meant to be frightening, and will fail on stage if it is not. All this gives us some justification for thinking of the theatre as less purely aesthetic than the other arts.

(Pole 1983: 13)

ADAPTIVE AND PATHOLOGICAL FORMS OF DETACHMENT

The above account has attempted to draw together the characteristics of aesthetic experience as defined by the artists. There is a strong suggestion of overlap and interrelatedness between aesthetic experience and the loss of ego identity during the state of depersonalisation. For example, aesthetic experience is described as involving a process of emotional disengagement. There is an interruption in the normal stream of consciousness. The sense of self is expedient, and is relegated to the background. The normal pattern of perception is altered so that the core experience takes place in context of personal abstraction.

In this sense, there are some similarities with the clinical concept of depersonalisation (see Chapter 6). However, the disengagement of which the aesthesticans talk is part of a heightened awareness and 'in-touchedness' with the percept, which feels 'mine', whereas depersonalisation comprises the converse. Whereas the aestheticians talk of loss or self capitulating to external stimuli for the achievement of sensual purity, the loss of identity in depersonalisation is a vacuum experience with no focus; rather than fascination, there is listlessness and a sense of having been locked outside the boundaries of one's own feeling. Instead of an enrichment of perception, events at the centre of consciousness seem unreal and remote.

Galdston (1947) took the view that in order to come to terms with the meaning of depersonalisation it is necessary to become acquainted with its opposite, a state which he termed 'personalisation'. Unfortunately, he did not go on to define the concept he created, but it is legitimate in this context to reflect on experiences brought about by transcendental meditation (TM). The meditative state has special phenomenological qualities, which are distinctive enough to merit a separate category within the area of psychic functioning. Successful participants in TM report a greater reinforcement of identity, and a feeling of unity between inner being and the external environment. In essence, TM usually generates a state corresponding to 'personalisation'. However, TM, as with any other technique which produces substantial changes in quality of consciousness, can sometimes generate unpleasant side-effects. Interestingly, casualties of the approach sometimes experience distressing feelings of unreality.

Kennedy (1976) was impressed by this; he noted that while successful participants acquire an enlightened experience, unsuccessful participants complain of sensations identical to depersonalisation. Rather than assume that TM precipitates correspondingly different states in different people, Kennedy attributes the variation in hedonic tone to differences in personal interpretation of the same basic experience:

> the intriguing aspect of [depersonalisation] is that apparently by using virtually the same mental maneuvers, depending on the attitude a person adopts towards himself and then towards the resulting phenomenon, may be experienced either as something to be sought and valued or something to be feared and called a disease. Perhaps what we ought to do with people who exhibit Primary Depersonalisation syndrome is to teach them first to accept themselves uncritically and, second, to accept their depersonalisation. Individuals who observe nonjudgementally do not describe their altered perceptions as flat and devoid of colour but as exhibiting increased colour.

> (Kennedy 1976)

When reading psychopathologists' accounts of depersonalisation phenomena, it is important to bear in mind that their view of this range of states is heavily coloured by the sample of the population with whom they deal. The clientele of the psychiatrist is not a happy one; if a person were content with his lot, he would be unlikely to consult the psychiatrist in the first place. Therefore, the psychiatric view of depersonalisation phenomena can only be biased, since it is based on the accounts of a non-random sample of people. If Kennedy's impressions are to be taken seriously, there are those content with their depersonalisation who are unlikely to seek help for an experience that they welcome. With particular reference to derealisation, this point is underlined by Skelton-Roberts (1975), who makes the following remarks:

> We note that depersonalisation is not always an unpleasant phenomenon. Some subjects are unterrified by their experiences, others find an element of positive excitement in the changes. As one dignified middle-aged matron said to us of

her experience of floating, 'I think this is what the hippies are trying to get'. Now this form of reaction plainly runs counter to our term affliction if we are to judge by experience alone.

(Skelton-Roberts 1975)

The implication of the accounts of both Kennedy and Skelton-Roberts is that there is considerable overlap between enhancement of perception and 'maladaptive' states of unreality.

What is acceptable to the aesthetician may be unacceptable to the clinician and vice versa. The relatedness between 'aesthetic' and 'clinically-defined' depersonalised states might prompt the reader to surmise that they represent good and bad aspects respectively of personal disengagement. Conceivably, these two experiences may lie at opposite ends of the same spectrum: a style of perception which is either potentially detrimental to or enhancing of life experience. It has been pointed out, for instance, that perception can be enriched or diminished by meditation techniques, implying that both perceptual modes share the same source, i.e. are precipitated by similar circumstances. Bearing in mind the possible relatedness, it may be more than mere coincidence that while the aestheticians suggest that women are more amenable than men to the aesthetic mode (Pole 1983), the psychiatrists point to a similar gender bias in the depersonalised mode (Sedman 1970). In short, there may be a tendency for the same population to be more sensitive to both modes, perhaps as a result of the adoption of a particular style of perception, the hedonic tone of which can vary.

It is difficult to anticipate whether such speculation has any repercussions within the fields from which the two concepts of aesthetic experience and depersonalisation emanate, i.e. theoretical aesthetics and clinical psychiatry. For the aesthetician, reflection on the properties of depersonalisation may help further sharpen up the definition of aesthetic experience, by the process of exclusion. For the psychiatrist, though he may be bemused by the suggestion, it may prove productive to acknowledge the similarity in quality between the problem his patient presents in the clinic, and the pleasure that the art appreciator derives from the gallery. Moreover, the enjoyment that some subjects report in association with depersonalisation suggests that the state should not be automatically categorised as maladaptive; enjoyable forms of depersonalisation bear a striking resemblance to aesthetic experience and exhibit an intrinsically-aesthetic quality.

The art gallery and concert hall seem a long way from the psychiatric clinic, but can we confidently say that the psychological hallmark of each is so drastically different? In treatment, perhaps it may be possible to manipulate depersonalisation and harness it to good effect, as, it seems, some subjects are capable of doing in day-to-day life.

Finally, the issues raised might encourage more conservative clinicians to re-evaluate their view of depersonalisation, in the light of its potentially enlightening underbelly. To deny the potential value of this experiential area may have ominous practical and theoretical repercussions, both for the aesthetician and the psychiatric patient. To underline this point, the following is an extract from a clinical thesis:

> where abnormal experiences of the ego are presented to us as enjoyable, this pleasure cannot alter the criterion of our judgement. We are not hedonists and we do not judge the worth of a thing by the satisfaction it affords. From our point of view the phenomenon of depersonalisation is identical whether there is pleasure or terror in reaction of the subject. Depersonalisation is not a potentiation or development of self but a disruption. The self is not carried further as an entity but is dislocated through its own mechanics. Therefore the term affliction is justified even in those cases where the disorder affords an element of satisfaction.
>
> (Skelton-Roberts 1975)

Such an emphatic statement may inadvertently discourage patients' successful efforts to shrug off maladaptive aspects of their own depersonalisation. Also, might not such a philosophically-arrogant assertion, however well-intentioned, intrude upon the private world of aesthetic experience itself, and attempt to police it?

SUMMARY

There is as yet no clear definition of 'ideal' states, emotions, perceptual style or cognitive style that can be viewed as the antagonists of maladaptive experience. Aesthetic experience, nirvana and flow experiences, and peak experience share a common denominator, in that they are all states of ego-enhancement. Each of these special states has a specific subjective quality, and serves a different purpose, determined by the philosophical orientation on which it is based. However, they share in common an ecological referent, in that they are all experiences that occur in relation to a self-world context. Phenomenological study of these various ideal states, to the same level of sophistication as psychopathological states, is highly desirable. The analysis should be couched in the same terms of reference as aberrant psychological phenomena. This is important in so far as ideal experiences may clarify the direction in which adaptive change due to therapeutic manoeuvres can be best effected.

The concept of aesthetic experience is particularly interesting in that there is some estrangement of the ego, in the sense that the subject reports feeling abstracted from the self. Some theorists question whether estrangement of the ego is necessarily unhealthy, pointing to examples of ego-detachment that generate a sense of enlightenment. The differential role of feeling states and heightened awareness is unclear. Many art philosophers suggest that a diminished awareness of self and a reduction in self-reflective thinking enhance the clarity of the external percept. It is argued that the diminution of awareness of self is only possible when the subjective conditions involve a reduced intensity of emotional output.

Chapter 10

Some common ground between phenomenological and cognitive psychology

ISSUES OF 'EXPLANATION': STATIC AND GENETIC UNDERSTANDING

In Chapter 1, Jaspers's two senses of the term 'understanding' (static and genetic) were discussed. To recap, static understanding refers to the analysis of experience within a momentary time-frame, irrespective of the temporal sequence of psychological events in which it is embedded, while genetic understanding is concerned with experience in the context of a causal sequence. Static analysis is concerned with the meaning of experience, as it is occurring, and corresponds to Heidegger's (1927) concept of *Dasein-analysis*. The differentiation of the description of the here-and-now distressing events and a temporal analysis of distress-inducing events is not new to clinical psychology and is reflected in behaviour therapy, for example, by Kanfer and Phillips's (1970) differentiation between functional and topographic aspects of a problem in behaviour therapy.

Topographic data relate to the overt features of a problem as exhibited by the patient. Functional aspects, on the other hand, relate to variables which are in some way causally related. Functional information is illuminated by the therapist's behavioural formulation of the problem, usually couched within a learning-theory paradigm. A functional level of analysis reflects hypotheses of underlying processes, particularly environmental and interoceptive cues, the effects of which are explained in terms of the subject's history of reinforcement. It is the postulation of underlying processes (albeit from a subjective source) which is most closely related to the phenomenological concept of 'genetic explanation'.

The subject matter of psychopathology involves complex sequences of events, so that a variety of factors, including environmental events, data from memory and distinct emotional states interact. Where there is a sequence of internal and external events leading to the symptomatology, the terms 'aetiology' and 'cause' should be modified to read 'aetiological sequence' or 'causal chain'.

A value of static phenomenological research is that, in carrying out a *Dasein-analysis*, the clinician can be discriminating in identifying the components of a given clinical presentation before going on to acquire a genetic understanding of the problem. In the current text, the relationship between a static and genetic mode of analysis is exemplified by Beck (1976) and Rapee (1986) respectively. Beck emphasised the process of catastrophisation in the here-and-now experience of panic, characterised by the overwhelming flood of dread and helplessness that accompanies thoughts of despair and the expectation of total incapacity. Beck illustrated a psychological state of affairs comprising the nature of the panic experience, the construction of which is achieved by the dissection of panic attacks as they occur, rather than examining the possible mechanisms which may have engendered the panic state.

Rapee (1985), on the other hand, approached panic from a genetic perspective, in the Jasperian sense, examining the possible precursors and consequences of the panic state. Rapee compared baseline heart and respiration rate in anxiety versus panic-disorder patients. These baseline measures were taken during periods that the patients judged as being 'safe', that is, a period of relative security in which they were symptom-free of acute distress. Rapee found that during these baseline periods, the respiration and heart-rate of panic patients was much higher than that of anxiety patients, suggesting that even minor upward shifts in the physiological pattern would form vivid interoceptive sensations difficult to accommodate.

In a subsequent experiment, Rapee *et al.* (1986) found that panic patients did not panic during periods of guided hyperventilation, largely because the resulting interoceptive sensations could be meaningfully linked by the patient to the respiration change and were therefore not construed as threatening. Rapee *et al.* therefore concluded that conditions generating panic arose due to changes in interoceptive sensation, but only when the genesis of the sensation was poorly understood (see Chapter 4). Rapee's 'genetic' research followed on from Beck's static conception of panic, without which Rapee's research strategy is unlikely to have been developed.

THE THEORETICAL STATUS OF SCHEMATA IN PROMOTING 'GENETIC EXPLANATION'

Schemata form a concept that forges links between cognitive science (as the science of human information processing) and what the clinician observes. Schemata are inferred organisational structures which guide experience by influencing the focus of awareness. According to Beck *et al.* (1990), schemata activate stored material, selectively cueing emotional, cognitive and behavioural data. Though they exhibit some consistency through time, schemata have dynamic properties, in the sense that they can shift in prominence and level of activation. The valency of a schema may fluctuate, so that its influence on information processing varies accordingly. Schemata are thought to 'jostle' one another into position, so that a schema which at a given moment is hypervalent will excite and inhibit other schemata selectively. Schemata influence 'being-in-the-world' from start to finish, in that they

(1) determine attentional bias, and thus the content of data central to awareness;
(2) determine how the attended percept is construed and interpreted;

(3) shape the response to the interpretation by schematically-organised planning, particularly schemata which pertain to the range of instrumental plans.

Beck et al. (1990) suggest that schemata can either be latent, that is, have no influence on current view of the world, or activated, in which case appraisal is biased in the direction of the schematic theme. When maladaptive schemata are activated, they displace and inhibit more adaptive appraisal, introducing a systematic bias into information processing. Consequently, there is a loss of reality-testing ability. As a technical term, schemata refers both to structural properties, in the form of a grouping together of propositional information, and to a process, engaging in the active selection and interpretation of the constant flow of incoming information. Beck et al. (1990) observe that subjects are unaware of their own schemata. For example, Beck has suggested that dizziness shares a meaningful connection with an anticipation of loss of balance and anticipation of unsteady gait. For Beck (1990), the phobic reaction to bridges and high places is an extension of fears of falling. It is feasible that dizziness prompts a change in body schema, producing a shift in attentional bias towards situations in which it would be dangerous to be disoriented in three-dimensional space, despite the fact that the disorientation is anticipated rather than real. Many patients do not appreciate the link between their dizzy symptoms and fear of heights until the implicit assumptions and predictions of their own behaviour are fully explored.

An important issue with which Beck's cognitive model needs to contend is an account of how schemata change from having little effect on awareness, as 'pre-potent' (Beck et al. 1990: 33), to becoming 'hypervalent', that is, having a strong influence on information-processing. Beck distinguishes between cognitive and affective types of schemata on the basis that 'the cognitive schemas are concerned with abstraction, interpretation, and recall; the affective schemas are responsible for the generation of feelings' (Beck et al. 1990: 33). The relationship between cognitive and affective schemata is reflected by the work of such authors as Velten (1968) and Gilligan and Bower (1984), outlined in Chapter 2. These authors have investigated the effects of thought on feeling and vice versa. Since there was internal consistency between the content or theme of each of the verbal and affective aspects of experience in these experiments, their work can be seen as early attempts to activate and manipulate schemata, and examine the effect of cognitive and affective shemata on each other.

Not all cognitive psychologists are satisfied with the notion of schemata, arguing that they are not sufficiently rigorous as theoretical constructs. The validation of schemata is in its infancy, and may await a clear procedure for the identification of schemas and their measurement. Lee (1992) has written critically about cognitive-therapy and in the process complained about the vagueness of cognitive-therapy concepts. She argues that cognitive schemas are merely hypothetical constructs about parsimonious themes in self-reporting. Many cognitive concepts, she claims, are little more than metaphors, labelling process variables without explaining their holistic functional roles. This vagueness means that it is impossible to predict cognitive activity at any given moment, nor how schemas from different sources will interact. Of course, when considering the interaction of schemas, it is essential to discriminate between one schema and another, procedural guidelines for which await models of schematic organisation. Various models are beginning to emerge, but are some way from being fully established. There has been a recent trend to view schemas as dynamic and interactive in their development and function. That is, schemas are high-order patterns of connections, controlling the selective activation of stored data for consciousness. Can schemas be segregated?

Teasdale and Barnard (1993) have attempted to partition emotional and 'cognitive' schemas by mode. Teasdale (1993) suggests that though the semantic schemas give meaning to events, generic emotional codes of an implicational nature generate fundamental intuitions, such as 'something is wrong', or 'I'm on the right track'. Contradicting the *force majeure* of most contemporary hypotheses, Teasdale accords priority-of-awareness to an unanalytical schema over cognitive schema which subsequently effect critical evaluation. The intuitive feeling of suspiciousness that often precedes the onset of a paranoid psychosis fits this level of functioning; there is no particular propositional self-statement of any substance accompanying the suspiciousness, apart from the vague reflection that something is not as it should be and that it is therefore necessary to be on guard against becoming the victim of unexpected and intentional harm. The intuition is otherwise unfocussed.

In many ways, Teasdale's view represents a throwback to Zajonc's (1984) affective primacy hypothesis. Recently, further attempts to clarify the role of unattached emotion have been carried out. Murphy and Zajonc (1993) presented either a smiling face (positive emotional priming) or a scowling face (negative emotional priming) before presenting a series of emotionally-benign Chinese ideographs selected for their novelty, ambiguity and blandness. The subjects were then asked to rate the idiographs on a like/dislike dimension of preference. They found that when the faces were presented for a period long enough for subjects to become aware of the facial percept, they had little effect in priming preference. However, when the faces were presented subliminally, scowling faces were followed by a net negative preference for the subsequently presented ideograph, while subliminally-presented smiling faces were followed by preferential ratings of the same stimuli.

Murphy and Zajonc (1993) suggest that subliminal perception bypasses linguistic processing and leads to the selective excitation of feeling states, at a barely conscious, preverbal level, and cite their results as evidence that affective memories influence subsequent evaluative decisions in a mood-congruent direction. Their results are consistent with the findings of Gilligan and Bower (1984) that provocation of specific affect shapes the subject's assessment of events.

Teasdale (1993) suggests that schemata are not connections of isolated thoughts or feelings, but form an interrelated network, which processes data for its significance and implications. Hence, he suggests that cognitive therapy should concentrate less on invalidating the client's isolated, negative automatic thoughts, and pay more attention to replacing higher-level implicational codes with alternative patterns of networking. For example, he suggests that changes at the 'implicational level' of processing occur at an earlier stage of lowered affect, when there is a minor mood change. This minor affective shift is thought to excite a network of schemata, from cognitive, affective and motor schemas. Teasdale therefore suggests that behavioural interventions, aimed at changing body posture and facial expression, should supplement therapies that engage the linguistic mode, in line with the observations of Ekman and Auster (1979) that nonverbal behaviours are causally related to affect, as independent variables of mood. The effect of experiential techniques which are nonverbal is, according to Teasdale, demystified by their integration into his information-processing model (Teasdale 1993).

The idea of separate schemas for emotion and verbal cognition has been pursued by Greenberg and Safran (1987). They argue that psychotherapeutic strategies must deal separately with affect resolution, and suggest a series of exercises based on gestalt notions of 'going for the feel', i.e. tuning in specifically to diffuse emotional experience and deliberately avoiding any interpretation. Attempts to adjust verbal propositions are likely to be unsuccessful or only partially effective unless affective schemata are contiguously 're-wired' into linguistic propositional networks. Verbally-mediated tasks are used later to re-frame approaches to emotionally-laden situations, but there has to have been a prior affective component attached to the adaptive propositional thought for it to be effective when the emotion reoccurs, giving the affect meaning and substance. The separation of emotional and cognitive schemas is supported by experiments on emotional suppression, which suggest that emotional experience remains similar even if its expression is inhibited at a linguistic level (Gross and Levenson 1993). We would like to add that, though the direction of this research is an interesting one, there is some conceptual confusion in the way in which these authors use the terms 'cognition' and 'emotion'. The gist of the argument which Teasdale (1993) and Gross and Levenson (1993) put forward is that it is useful for the client to access maladaptive feeling states, at a fairly undifferentiated level, before an adaptive reinterpretation of those states can be effectively brought about linguistically.

Safran (1990) defines a schema as a programme for maintaining relatedness with the world, which contains tacit rules, but not necessarily bits of concrete information. A key point of Safran's model is that schemas are actively constituted and maintained by self-fulfilling loops, rather than stored as representations. The closed nature of schemas makes them difficult to access therapeutically and, according to Safran, this difficulty results from the dynamics of an interpersonal loop that becomes self-perpetuating, as a style of relating to the world. The individual shapes his or her world by construing and constructing it. Rigidity of schemas is revealed in a fixed pattern of feelings and response dispositions as well as the way the client reports them. Safran suggests that a key factor in modifying closed schemas is modifying the communication of the client. In such manipulations, the therapist plays the role of 'unhooking' the person from the schematic cycle by changing self-perpetuating interpretations by the subject.

Safran's conception of schemas as self-perpetuating loops draws the history of schemata full circle, towards a phenomenological perspective in that schema are defined as how the person relates to the world in the here and now. Schema are not seen as stored representations, suspended in an ambiguous juxtaposition to conscious awareness, but as dynamic patterns, continually activated and re-activated in the present by a cognitive interpersonal cycle. In the clinical context, Safran's aim is to distance the patient from the self-maintenance of maladaptive schemas by focusing on details of interactive style with the therapist. The approach mirrors the phenomenological method of changing awareness by detached description of a thought pattern. But there is a crucial difference between the phenomenological and Safran's approach, in that Safran is uncritical in his approach to considering the profile of assumptions (schemas) of the observer or the therapist, and there is a tendency in his model to assume that the therapist can interpret the client's behaviour without imposing biased interpretive meaning.

Georgi (1992), in a recent article comparing description and interpretive strategies in exposing meaning, notes that description involves the clarification of meaning of experience as experienced. Interpretation is the clarification of the meaning of an experience in terms of plausible assumptions. The descriptive scientist believes that meaning can be teased out by describing meaning precisely as it presents itself. In a comment that could be addressed directly to Safran, Georgi asks why the therapist should force a closure on something that announces itself as non-closed. His point is that the seeking of possible orderings between thoughts and emotions, where in fact there is only an ambiguity in this order, is what transforms the analytic situation from a descriptive to an interpretive one. If schema are interpretations, their ambiguities, which cause the client conflict and maladaptation, may be better revealed by a descriptive analysis rather than by yet more interpretation from the therapist.

SCHEMATA AND CHILDHOOD AETIOLOGY

Most therapists, whatever their persuasion, acknowledge that quality of childhood experience, reflected by such things as degree of parental support, exposure to adaptive role models and consistency of warm, supportive relationships are important predictors of later adjustment (Van der Kolk *et al.* 1991). The traditional strategy of psychoanalysis comprises the re-exposure of early events in consciousness, with a view to further retrospective self-evaluation and reassessment of current self-understanding. The psychoanalytic model assumes that distress is largely the product of repressed memories pertaining to early childhood experiences; corrective intervention lies in exploring memories, often barely accessible, pertaining to events in the remote past. Recently, cognitive theorists have began to reconsider the mechanisms by which early traumatic events influence current thinking and behaviour. A crucial question being asked is how the effects of early maladaptive experience are transmitted over time, so that these early experiences have a detrimental effect on current psychosocial adaptability?

It has been proposed that some pathogenic schemata are formed early in life and are constructed by the subject to reflect experience, in the form of core assumptions and expectations. At least some of these core beliefs are thought to be resistant to modification over time and have been termed Early Maladaptive Schemata. The notion of Early Maladaptive Schemata (EMSs) is fairly recent (Young 1990). EMSs are said to influence current functioning in that the core beliefs of which they consist are implicated in the elicitation of negative automatic thoughts (Layden et al. 1993). Layden et al. suggest that the content of an individual's schemata can be roughly demarcated on the basis of his/her themes of behaviour and negative automatic thinking, in the form of a 'cognitive response set' (our term) and is conceptually related to the notion of a construct system, by which relatively stable views of the world are organised (Kelly 1955). This cognitive organisation is thought to bias appraisal of information, and information attended to, so that EMSs have a major impact on psychosocial development.

The notion of transmission of early traumatic experience in the form of a perceptual-evaluative style is a deterministic view of human development, which is likely to encourage therapists to consider the formation of early, self-maintaining construct systems. The implication for therapy is an important one: unlike psycho-analysis, the effects of early experience on current existence are seen in terms of information-processing bias, rather than personality dynamics. The lasting effects of sexual abuse, which are all too obvious throughout the lives of many patients, can often be viewed as the manifestations of persistent schema structures, oriented around the perceived degree of instrumental control at the time of the abuse and the untrustworthiness of adults of the same gender as the abuser.

SCHEMATA AND ATTENTIONAL BIAS DURING INFORMATION-SEEKING

With regard to bias in appraisal of the world, there is evidence to suggest that cognitive bias is not only linked to evaluation of data in consciousness; evidence from clinical subjects suggests that distortions also occur in the content of the data to be evaluated. Much of the research related to this area has been derived from the measurement of attentional focus of subjects asked to name colours on a modified form of the Stroop test. The modified Stroop test consisted of a number of phobia-related words, each written in a different colour. The task involved naming the colour of each word, thus focusing attention on the colour rather than the printed word. Literate adults have a tendency to read the word rather than name its colour and therefore there is an experimental conflict of investment of attention. Perfor-mance on the Stroop is measured by reaction time in colour-naming. The longer the time taken to name the colour of each word, the more powerfully the subject's attention is distracted to the word itself. Watts et al. (1986) compared the reaction time of arachnophobics and controls in colour-naming printed words when the words themselves were spider-related. They found that the spider-phobic group took longer to name the colours of the spider-related words than non-phobic subjects. Watts *et al.* went on to re-test the phobic subjects following treatment and found that the successfully-desensitised subjects exhibited a much improved reaction time. The results suggest that when there is an emotional investment in a specific theme (in this case, fear and spiders), there is a greater readiness to attend to theme-related aspects of a stimulus than to theme-unrelated aspects.

Mathews and MacLeod (1985) attributed similar findings in the relationship between phobic anxiety and Stroop-test performance to the greater degree of attentional investment in the meaning of the words themselves compared with colour recognition, or, alternatively, to the interference of colour-recognition performance by increased arousal, elicited by fear-related words but not neutral words. Mathews and MacLeod compared colour-naming reaction time of two types of untreated anxiety patients and non-anxious controls. The anxious patients were divided into those with hypochondriacal preoccupation and those with predominantly social anxiety. Compared with the controls, anxious patients as a whole exhibited retarded colour-naming of words related to negative social performance, such as 'pathetic' and 'inadequate'. Hypochondriacal subjects, but neither the controls nor patients prone to social anxiety, exhibited significantly slower naming of the colours of health-related words (e.g. 'deathbed'). For a succinct discussion on these experiments in attentional bias, see Brewin (1988: 71–74).

The above data supports the notion that attentional mechanisms edit perceptual input by ushering the patient towards danger signals, safe signals having a greater latency of recognition. The effect of schemata on attentional bias is an important one, though research in this area may be hampered by the operational definition of schemata and, related to this, the consensus of opinion across clinicians evaluating schematic organisation of the same patient. If the identification of schemata has low inter-rater reliability because of the arbitrarily-defined boundaries in cognitive organisation, predictive studies of EMSs, for example, will be difficult. It is questionable whether a procedure will be developed by which schemata can be reliably identified across clinicians. Schemata are statistical abstractions, in that schemata are the product of cluster analyses, however informally carried out, of surface cognitions, and are therefore accessed in the clinical situation by verbal report. Therapist bias in the identification of schemata is extremely likely, and variability in clinical judgement by different clinicians evaluating the same patient is an important shortcoming. It may well be that the schemata which the therapist constructs of his own patients is a compromise position, shared by patient and therapist, which is the evaluative interface between what the patient says and the schemata that the therapist brings with him or her to the session. Perhaps schemata could be operationally defined by attentional bias, as in the Stroop experiment above.

SOME RECENT PSYCHOLOGICAL PERSPECTIVES ON DELUSIONS

Defining delusions

In the strict phenomenological sense, there is no such thing as a delusion, since there is no such thing as a false belief from a purely subjective point of view. To the beholder, a belief is simply a reflection of reality as he or she sees it, whether or not it is evaluated as false by others. Phenomenology is the study of subjective activity, while the judgement of erroneousness is made on objective grounds. As Sims puts it:

> There can be no phenomenological definition of delusion, because the patient is likely to hold this belief with the same conviction and intensity as he holds other non-delusional beliefs about himself; or as anyone else holds intensely personal non-delusional beliefs. Subjectively, a delusion is simply a belief.
>
> (Sims 1988: 84)

Nonetheless, on pragmatic grounds, most clinical phenomenologists use the term delusion to indicate gross distortion in the assessment of external events, often to the extent that the subject's welfare is compromised.

Sims (1988) lists three defining characteristics of delusions as:

1   ideas held with unusually strong conviction, which
2   are not amenable to logic, and
3   have an absurd or erroneous content, which is manifest to others.

An important distinction is made between primary and secondary delusions (Cutting 1985; Sims 1988). Primary delusions arise spontaneously, with apparent discontinuity with preceding conscious activity. Primary delusions consist of propositional thoughts that have no discernible origin and are therefore 'un-understandable'. Secondary delusions can be linked to the presence of a pervasive mood state, such as nihilistic delusions in severe depression (see Chapter 4), or form the extension of a cultural belief. For an example of the latter, see Yap (1965) on Koro syndrome.

Phenomenological writers with extensive experience of deluded patients, such as Schneider (1959), Fish (1967) and Cutting (1985), have dissected the qualitative experiences of their deluded patients, deconstructing the progression of psychological events around which a primary delusion takes place. This has been done by observing patients during their deterioration and also from retrospective accounts, when the patients have regained full lucidity. There is general agreement among eminent psychopathologists that the development of delusional belief is preceded by a period in which the subject's world is pregnant with anticipation and shrouded in ambiguity (delusional atmosphere), accompanied by feelings of uncomfortable bewilderment or suspicion (delusional mood), sometimes of several months' duration. When the delusion arises, this state of tension terminates abruptly, as it is swept away by the overwhelming rush of apparent meaningfulness.

The moment at which the false unshakeable belief appears has been the focus of intense *Dasein-analysis*. This is an area in which cognitive psychologists are likely to become increasingly involved in the coming years. In particular, information processing at the moment of inception of delusional ideation is of considerable interest. One area of concern is exactly how a delusion crystallises out within the subjective conditions surrounding its birth. Schneider (1959) reflects that the essence of the experience is the reinterpretation of relatively benign external events, which are suddenly attributed profound significance. According to Schneider, there is no distortion of the incoming sensory data, so that sensory percepts remain unchanged. The change which occurs is *evaluative* in nature, so that the same percepts representing external stimuli are invested with an intuitive feeling of vital significance, and are construed by the subject as possessing immense personal implications for the patient.

Traditionally, many phenomenologists have regarded most delusions to be impenetrable because of their fixedness. However, Garety (1985) and Walkup (1990) have challenged the idea that delusions remain fixed and incorrigible over time. Garety (1985) constructed statements for each of her two deluded subjects which were representative of their delusional beliefs and requested them to indicate their extent of agreement (as a measure of degree of conviction), on a weekly basis. She found that the degree of conviction fluctuated. For some cognitive therapists, the malleability of delusional intensity signifies that psychological manipulation of delusional beliefs is more realistic a task than their earlier phenomenological colleagues assumed.

In a sample of nine schizophrenic in-patients, Brett-Jones, Garety and Hemsley (1987) confirmed fluctuations in the conviction with which delusions were held, and observed that a decrease in conviction predicted the subsequent amount of time thinking about the delusion itself. This suggests that conviction is a valid and quick barometer of flexibility in the mental state, with potential implications for the timing of treatment attempting to regulate delusional thinking.

SOME COMMENTS ON COGNITIVE RESEARCH RELATED TO DELUSIONS

Cognitive psychologists are beginning to make some interesting contributions to the measurement and management of psychotic phenomena, a field to which the psychiatry profession has previously had an almost exclusive involvement. Much of this work has been directed towards process research. Some of the research aims are consistent with the phenomenological concept of 'genetic understanding', in converging on a particular characteristic of psychotic patients and teasing out its experiential components. One notable example is the work of Garety and colleagues (1991), who have studied problem-solving strategies of deluded patients, in order to shed light on delusion-formation. The experimental paradigm consisted of presenting deluded patients with a task requiring probabilistic judgements over a period of time in which heuristic information was introduced progressively. The task involved guessing throughout the procedure whether the majority of balls in an opaque jar were black or white in colour, and the subjects were informed at the outset that one-third of the balls were of one colour and two-third of the other. The jar was emptied of the balls one at a time. Irrespective of how many balls of each colour were eventually extracted from the jar, the deluded subjects tended to persist with their initial hypothesis, in contrast to non-deluded controls, whose estimation of majority colour changed heuristically, depending on the proportion of black or white balls eventually extracted.

Garety *et al.* (1991) concluded that while controls demonstrated flexibility of hypotheses-formation according to the data presented, deluded subjects remained fixated on their original hypothesis, regardless of whether it was contradicted through subsequent evidence, a phenomena which Garety *et al.* described as premature, perseverative 'jumping to conclusions'. The potential significance of such a finding may become more apparent if it is firmly established that, in everyday life situations, the normal population is prone to bizarre thoughts, perhaps largely of a fleeting nature, which are immediately disregarded in the light of counter-information. Garety's work would suggest that deluded people fail to suspend validation of such hypotheses, until further confirmatory or disconfirmatory evidence is obtained, jumping to conclusions prematurely and failing to modify those conclusions in the light of fresh evidence.

It remains to be seen whether the same 'jumping to conclusions' mechanism is implicated in delusional perception. It is feasible, for example, that we all form 'crazy, high-risk' hypotheses, but that in delusion-free subjects, these hypotheses stay in consciousness only fleetingly in the face of contrary evidence. Delusion-prone subjects, on the other hand, may cling to 'high risk' hypotheses, which become delusions because they 'stick', becoming core beliefs.

An example of adaptive, flexible hypotheses-testing is illustrated by an experience of one of the current authors, who, when crossing a T-junction on foot, was startled by the sight of a car cornering at speed. For a fleeting moment, he held the notion that the car was deliberately swerving into his path; that the driver was aiming the vehicle intentionally at him, the potential victim. As he stepped back to the curb, the car sped past, leaving the shaken pedestrian looking on, cursing the driver for recklessly careless, rather than homicidal driving. Since the driver did not alter course as the pedestrian made his escape, the idea of homicidal intent was immediately forgotten; given the tendency for deluded patients to retain initial hypotheses in the face of contrary evidence, it is not difficult to see how transitory hypotheses, in this case of a suspicious flavour, might persist, forming a paranoid delusion. The role of the 'jumping to conclusions' process in delusional perception has not as yet been fully ascertained, but may go some way to explain the conviction that patients portray in secondary delusions, but not primary delusions, which are bizarre and apparently unrelated to prior events.

Schematic organisation accompanying delusions

Cognitive schemas reflect an individual's overall view of the world. This world-view inevitably incorporates general assumptions and abstractions, including cause-effect relationships, particularly with regard to their significance to the subject. The judgemental patterns concerning causation form the 'attributional style' of the subject. Bentall *et al.* (1994) claim to have identified a distinct attributional style portrayed by deluded subjects. Bentall suggests that while depressed subjects attribute all good external events to outside agencies and all negative events to themselves, paranoid subjects have a tendency to attribute all good events to themselves and all negative events to outside agencies. The evidence for this conclusion is based on an experimental procedure in which two criterion groups, of paranoid patients and depressed patients, were presented with a series of hypothetical positive and negative events (Kaney and Bentall 1989). Subjects were then asked to judge the underlying causes of these events. The depressed patients tended to attribute bad events to themselves and good events to other influences, indicating a 'good-for-nothing' self-image, in which self is perceived as being of detrimental value. Conversely, the paranoid subjects demonstrated the tendency to attribute bad events to others and good events to themselves: 'life would be fine if it wasn't for other people'.

The results of the above experiment were replicated by Candido and Romney (1990), who included depressed patients, paranoid patients and, in addition, patients exhibiting both features simultaneously. The clinical criteria of each mental state was determined by self-rating scales, including the Beck Depression Inventory for the measurement of affective disorder (Beck *et al.* 1961) and the Maine Scale to measure paranoia (Vojtisek 1976). The Attributional Style Questionnire (Peterson *et al.* 1982) was also administered. This is a sixty-item scale which records and quantifies subjects' assessment of attributed causes attached to a series of positive and negative outcomes, which refer largely to everyday situations. Candido and Romney's data raises not only the question of the potential role of these two states (paranoia and depression), but also the wider question of how the two states interact with each other. We know that affective states shape information-processing events, to the extent that propositional thoughts 'fall into line' with the predominant affect (see Gilligan and Bower 1984; Chapter 2). The relationship between affect and cognition becomes more complex when there are two affective components which are present simultaneously. Do two sets of cognitions emerge, which correspond to their respective feeling states, or does a compromise cognitive pattern emerge, which in effect is a product of an affective mix? Candido and Romney were therefore interested in the attributional style of subjects in whom a mixture of affects occurs, forming a state of affairs sometimes described as an emotional 'palette' (Plutchick 1980; see Chapter 3). Their findings suggest that while this 'palette' group fell between the paranoid subjects and depressed subjects in the evaluation of positive events, bad events were evaluated in a style typical of paranoid subjects. The implications of these findings are unclear, but may suggest the dominance of one affect over another, only when the hedonic tone of the subject matter is negative.

In investigating the group of subjects with both paranoid and depressive features, the research raises the question of how the two states influence propositional thinking. For example, do paranoia and depression compete with each other, the type of attributional cognition corresponding to the more pronounced state dominating evaluative judgement, or do coexisting states generate a mid-line, consensus proposition? A fuller empirical investigation could be carried out on Romney and Candido's (1990) data, comparing the relative strength of paranoid and depressive features for each patient and examining the relation between relative scores and frequency of attribution. However, the data suggest that there may be a different process occurring in the effect of mood in assessed attribution for good events than there is for bad events. The influence of emotional 'palettes' on other schemas is as yet largely uninvestigated.

Both Candido and Romney (1990) and Bentall *et al.* (1994) imply that paranoia and depression are related phenomena, which do not arise from two different feeling states, but a single dysphoric mood, the quality of which varies according to attributional style. This view emphasises the importance of cognitive schemata in activating systematic attributional patterns and has important implications for a theory of schemata: the quality of abnormal experience is seen by the above authors as determined by linguistic rather than affective schemata, since the quality of emotion is described in terms of the subject's pattern of evaluative judgement, rather than the activation of primary affects. This theoretical view is a clear departure from Zajonc's (1984) 'affective primacy' hypothesis. For example, paranoia is seen not as a special affective schema, but a product of dysphoric affect, which takes on a more specific quality once judgements about the *meaning* of negative and positive events is made.

Candido and Romney (1990) suggest that paranoid delusions may be amenable to cognitive therapy, so long as the general attributional set, rather than the paranoid delusion itself, is confronted. Attempts to alter attributional style have been suggested by a number of authors, with some claims to success (see, for example, Fowler and Morley 1989). Several authors have warned that a direct confrontation with the deluded patient, pointing out the erroneous nature of his or her delusional beliefs, is ill-advised. A confrontational approach serves only to alienate the patient and sabotage rapport, since ideas and assumptions fundamental to the patient's current view of the world are undermined. Another shortcoming of making direct challenges of this nature is that the therapist is in danger of becoming integrated into the delusional belief, often as an agent of deliberate disinformation. However, changes in attributional style can be effected without choosing events central to delusional content, by training in re-attribution of good and bad events which are not involved in the delusional system of the patient, forming 'neutral territory' in which to work.

Problems of rapport between deluded patients and clinicians are common, but in most cases, these are not insurmountable. In a recent article, Alford and Beck

(1994) consider the use of cognitive therapy for delusional beliefs. The emphasis of this article is not so much on direct attempts at manipulating delusions, but on the issue of avoiding confrontation and establishing a working relationship. A question which as yet remains unanswered is the timing of intervention; given that delusional conviction fluctuates over time, it would be useful for cognitive therapists working in this area to know if there is an optimal time to intervene with therapeutic procedures. The common-sense view is presumably that the lower the degree of conviction, the more amenable the deluded patient will be to reorganise the evaluation of his/her world. Whether encouraging the patient to challenge a delusional belief during periods of relatively low levels of conviction reduces the maintenance of delusional activity in the longer term remains to be tested.

Psychologists often argue that it is unproductive to regard delusions as un-understandable, claiming that it is useful, in building a meaningful relationship with the patient, to attempt to forge links between delusional content and past experiences which may have led to the patient's particular style of erroneous thought. Though the content of thinking in delusions can sometimes be traced to issues with which the patient has been preoccupied, by virtue of life style or history, a major issue regarding delusional belief relates to form. Sims (1988) illuminates the issue by a case illustration, involving a middle-aged spinster who is convinced that she is anaesthetised by men who break into her flat and sexually molest her. He comments:

> We can understand, on obtaining more details of the history, how her disturbance centres on sexual experience; why she should be distrustful of men; her doubts about her femininity; and her feelings of social isolation. However, the delusion, her absolute conviction that these things are happening to her, that they are true, is not understandable. The best we can do is to try and understand externally, without really being able to feel ourselves into her position, what she is thinking and how she experiences it. We cannot understand how such a situation could have developed.
>
> This is the core of a primary or autochthonous delusion; it is ultimately un-understandable.

> (Sims 1988: 85)

Garety's (1985) work on the tendency of deluded individuals to 'jump to conclusions' may shed some light on this issue of information processing during delusion formation. Assume that Sims's patient was prone to distorted ideas and fantasies about the threat posed to her by men, but normally modulated such thoughts by reference to previous experience. It may be that the same fleeting propositions were taken as literal fact once a jumping to conclusions pattern was in operation, particularly when this leads to subsequent attentional bias in search of ostensibly confirmatory evidence. Delusions are defined by duration and the conviction with which they are held, not by content alone.

In a recent review of psychological theories of delusions, Hingley (1992) makes the point that cognitive theories fail to deal with process variables that might explain the un-understandability of primary delusions and the phenomenon of delusional perception. However, the limitations of current knowledge in primary delusions may not be important from a pragmatic point of view in the treatment of delusions themselves. This is because, as Hingley (1992) puts it, delusions may owe their *maintenance* to 'the tendency to attend to confirmatory rather than disconfirmatory evidence'. It is in this area that evaluative judgement is important, in that distorted attributional style, described by Kaney and Bentall (1989) and Candido and Romney (1990), exposes the subject to propositional self-statements that confirm rather than disconfirm the original delusional belief. This must inevitably affect the subject's thinking on a schematic level and general attributional assumptions can be viewed as schemata in their own right.

Psychotic phenomena as the splitting of self from thought: auditory hallucinations

Most auditory hallucinations of which patients complain comprise 'hearing voices' and are therefore verbal hallucinations. These phenomena are commonly viewed in phenomenological circles as a disorder of the form of thought. In normal forms of thought, the cognitive activity is assessed by an individual as emanating from the subject's own consciousness, and the resulting percept is judged to be intero-ceptive, that is, the stimulus events are construed as internal events. The subject knows that his thoughts, perceptions and actions are his own, and percepts arising out of thinking activity are 'felt' as internal, cognitive activity and an aspect of subjective space. In verbal hallucinatory experiences, on the other hand, the subject feels that his/her cognitive activity is arising outside of subjective space. When thoughts are ascribed to an external source, the resulting percept is felt as an auditory hallucination in the form of voices from outside, so that thoughts appear to be 'spoken' by someone else and are 'heard'. These are passivity experiences. Sims (1988) writes:

> All passivity experiences falsely attribute functions to not self influences from outside, which are actually coming from inside the self. The experience of auditory hallucinations are confidently ascribed by the patient to sensory stimuli outside the self whereas, in fact, they arise inside self . . . however, it is the interviewer identifying an ego disturbance or disorder of the patient's experience of self; the patient complains of the upsetting content, not of the disordered form of self-experience.

(Sims 1988: 160)

Though cognitive theory has explored the subjective processes of anxiety and depression, problems concerning awareness of self-induced activity are less well researched within the cognitive framework. The phenomenon of psychotic aliena-tion of thought, in which one's own thoughts are not experienced as emanating from the self, are complex disturbances of self-awareness, in which there is the intuitive but false impression that one's own cognitive percepts are distal stimuli, await dissection by cognitive scientists. This special level of dysfunctional awareness, in which there is a failure of the subject to appreciate that thinking belongs to his/her own subjective space, is of major significance to relatively more severe and protracted mental-health problems.

Not all verbal hallucinations are passivity experiences, since some patients complain of hearing their own thoughts out loud. The subject knows that his or her thoughts are their own, but 'hears' them, during, before or after the thought is itself experienced in subjective space. This is known as 'thought echo', 'audible thoughts', or by the French term *'echoes de pensées'* (Fish 1967). In audible thinking, the patient's attribution remains intact, in that thinking is judged to be owned by the self, and is under self-control, but a percept of identical content to the thinking process is perceived as being located outside of subjective space and is a considerable source of irritation and distress (see Sims 1988: 119). Audible thoughts are not passivity experiences, since thinking processes are experienced as under self-control and self-direction. They are attributed to a subjective source, while the 'hearing voices' type of hallucinations are not. The term 'attribution' requires some clarification in the present sense. Though attribution normally refers to a consciously-considered formulation of cause-effect relations, it is unlikely that hallucinosis will be preceded by introspective deductive activity during which the source of verbal material is considered. In the passivity type of hallucinosis, the impression of externality is immediate and automatic: there is little evidence that the patient erects attributional hypotheses regarding the location of the percept at the onset of passivity-type hallucinatory experience.

There is often a great deal of soul-searching introspection accompanying audible thoughts. Sims (1988) describes the patient's inner world at such times in the following terms:

> The patient knows that they are his thoughts, yet hears them audibly either while he is thinking them, just before, or just after. . . . The patient may feel that his brain is replaced by cotton wool or convoluted rubber. His thoughts are jumbled, muzzy, vague, blurred: 'I try to part my way through them but they are like treacle and keep coming back and making me stick'.
>
> (Sims 1988: 119)

Verbal hallucinations, then, can be viewed as products of inner speech, which have a dysfunctional form so that the inner speech is perceived abnormally as voices-of-others or as audible rather than inaudible thoughts-from-within. Information-processing theories have supported the view that auditory hallucinations are the product of dysfunctional linguistic processing. The evidence that auditory verbal hallucinations involve inner speech is reflected by the fact that sub-vocal muscular activity coincides with both normal form of thought in controls and the experience of verbal hallucinations in some patients (Green and Kinsbourne 1990).

Bentall *et al.* (1988) argue that researchers should investigate the individual features of psychoses rather than be bound by diagnostic categories. This is because diagnoses, such as schizophrenia, are a collection of symptoms which, as a bundle of features, are too burdensome to be investigated simultaneously. There has been a recent resurgence of interest in verbal hallucinations within the field of cognitive neuropsychology. For example, Frith (1987) reiterates the view that verbal hallucinations are a dysfunction of the monitoring of thought. This view is consistent with the phenomenological concept of 'thought alienation', in which the hallucinating patient fails to grasp that the percept in consciousness has arisen from within personal subjective space. Conceptual developments relating to alienation of thinking have been hampered by the lack of a model of cognitive-linguistic functioning which outlines information-processing patterns in the normal form of thinking of non-clinical subjects. This shortfall in the literature is beginning to be rectified, notably by the notion of 'working memory' (Baddeley 1986). Baddeley's model suggests that thoughts resonate in phonological form and take on the characteristics of internal 'sounds', before their meaning and significance can be ascertained by the subject (the so-called 'phonological loop').

Attempts have been made to implicate the phonological loop in auditory hallucinations. From the limited data and line of enquiry so far, it would appear that there is little evidence that a dysfunction within the loop is responsible for hallucinations consisting of audible voices (David and Lucas 1993), though David (1994) claims to have demonstrated experimentally a link between the phonological loop and hallucinations comprising audible thoughts (thought echo) in a single subject. This area of research exemplifies attempts at the 'genetic understanding' of hallucinatory phenomena in terms of an information-processing model.

Disorders of the thinking process are widespread in long-term mental-health problems, and appear to cause considerable disruption to the patient's life. Sometimes, hallucinations are heard as commands which the patient feels some degree of compulsion to follow. How do individuals cope with their disordered thinking? In an extensive survey involving 200 schizophrenic patients living in the community, Carr (1988) investigated the patients' personal ways of coping with each of their problematic subjective experiences. One of these experiences was 'thought disturbance', defined as an affirmative response to the question 'Have there been times in the past year when you felt that your thinking was mixed up or not under your full control, or that you were not able to make sense of things?' (see Carr 1988: 342). The methods most commonly used by patients as strategies to cope with disturbances of thinking were 'passive diversion' (use of external stimuli as passive distraction, for example, listening to music, watching television), and physical inactivity, accompanied by a feeling of resignation in awaiting diminution of the disturbance. None of the patients attempted to problem-solve during thought disturbance, i.e. indicated the use of reasoning or concrete strategies of active self-manipulation, though a few attempted to concentrate on a topic or percept unrelated to this group of symptoms. The survey illuminates the difficulties that schizophrenic patients have in both coming to terms with and resolving problems related to thinking processes. Unfortunately, the survey did not discriminate between problematic thinking by form.

Some authors have attempted to draw functional links between depersonalisation and the intentionality during passivity experiences. In the latter, the qualifying 'as if' prefix in the proposition 'as if not me' is missing, and so the analogy takes on a literal meaning. A breakdown of the contrastive analysis between 'mine' and 'not mine' occurs, so that percepts become attributed to an external source. Percepts, for example, are 'seen' or 'heard' as originating in three-dimensional space. When percepts are attributed to an external source, they are defined as hallucinations. Depersonalisation is of particular interest in psychopathology since it occupies a position between full self-awareness and total breakdown in the discrimination between 'I' and 'not I'. In depersonalisation, all subjective experience is attributed firmly as 'belonging-to-me', but this (correct) attributional evaluation is not authenticated at a different level of awareness, possibly at a feeling level. It would be of great interest to compare depersonalisation with psychotic passivity of thinking, in terms of intentionality. A comparison may help clarify our understanding of psychotic phenomena. In depersonalisation, patients complain that the feeling quality of experience is missing, but all percepts are nonetheless identified as 'my own'. Depersonalisation leaves intact the contrastive analysis of percepts arising from distal stimuli and percepts arising out of internal events of thought and imagination. Some subjects exhibit both depersonalisation and auditory hallucinations. It would be interesting to obtain accounts of hallucinosis, and thinking during depersonalisation, from patients who experience both phenomena.

TEACHING PHENOMENOLOGY AS A CLINICAL ORIENTATION

A major pitfall in attempting the formulation of a presenting problem is the attribution of an experience to an event that is causally incompatible. For example, a diagnosis can never be used as an explanation of abnormal behaviour or a dysfunctional emotional state: it is illogical to suggest that a patient is fearful or exhibits bizarre behaviour 'because of schizophrenia', since the term schizophrenia is an abstract construct, not a psychological event. However, it would be phenomenologically acceptable to suggest that the patient was bizarre and fearful because s/he believed that s/he was being controlled by magical forces bent on her/his destruction, or because s/he could hear voices swearing and saying s/he must harm her/himself or others. Similarly, it would be logically incorrect to state that a patient was disinhibited or socially inappropriate 'because of a brain lesion'. Phenomenologically, the patient may be unable to resist powerful urges or may lack judgement of socially appropriate expression. That is not to say that there is no correlation between aberrant behaviour and organic dysfunction; it is a statistical fact that brain and behaviour are linked. It is important to emphasise that phenomenologists would not argue that organic brain disease and abnormal behaviour coexist by chance. However, any attempt to explain behaviour and psychological sequelae on the basis of organicity represents premature closure, for the two entities (CNS abnormality and behavioural aberration) are incompatible phenomena, mediated by intervening processes, the nature of which is the essence of phenomenological analysis.

In this respect, students of medicine, whether or not they have been acquainted with the philosophical issues surrounding clinical practice, tend to be particularly prone to making errors of logic, since the bulk of their training is couched in terms of physical pathology being causally connected to physical symptoms, a supposition acceptable to phenomenologists, since the boundaries of physicality have not been breached. However, to say that physical events *explain experiential change* is a different matter, deemed logically incorrect by virtue of the lack of correspondence between being and physical matter. Matter does not experience anything, though, by some *unknown means*, it gives rise to experience. Students of clinical psychology, on the other hand, have a grounding in the study of behaviour and environmental influences on existence. They too exhibit a tendency for premature closure and this is particularly true in constructing explanations of psychotic phenomena. Often, there is a tendency to 'explain' the content of delusions in terms of prior life events of the patient, but a failure to demonstrate why one individual may become deluded while another, with comparable exposure to life events, does not. The essence of the difficulty here lies in inattention to form and an overemphasis on content.

Phenomenology can be taught as an abstract philosophy (for example, Husserl's concept of essences) or as an applied human science (for example, Fish 1967). In the clinical context, phenomenology is an important branch of applied descriptive psychopathology, referring to the subjective aspects of aberrant experience. In clinical training, it is common to sidestep any substantial involvement with philosophical concepts and, instead, concentrate on the practical steps that facilitate empathy and understanding. There are some clinical teachers who may disagree with this view, on the basis that, by learning the philosophical position, the acquisition of clinical observational skills will automatically follow. We do not share the view that empathy can be achieved once the appropriate philosophical position has been imparted, but rather regard prior knowledge, particularly in current models of variation of the form of experience, as essential if good clinical practice is to be engendered.

There are several reasons for having misgivings and reservations regarding the value of pure philosophy alone. First, armchair philosophy does not lend itself easily to immediate interpretation in the clinically-pragmatic sense. A student with only a philosophical background in phenomenological principles may be at a loss to investigate the mental state of a distressed patient. Not only are tact and respect for the patient's defences a contextual skill, but the optimal tempo and linguistic style with which the clinician conducts an interview are developed through clinical experience. Second, patients often convey descriptions of their experiences couched in obscure terms and previous knowledge of psychopathology can greatly assist in elucidating the psychological events to which the patient is exposed. Prior knowledge of a framework by which to give structure to the form of self-report as well as elucidation of its content is essential. Third, the student's intellectual acquisition of a philosophical position does not necessarily lead to a reciprocal increase in assessment skills; a student may have a highly-developed axiomatic knowledge of principles, but be unable to 'live out' these principles in practice.

Existential psychology has a special value for cognitive theorists who take into consideration severe mental-health problems. The psychoses, in particular, have been relatively less explored by psychopathologists of a cognitive persuasion than by other psychopathologists. While cognitive theorists have been well established in the area of experiences of self which are of positive amplitude, those of negative amplitude, in which there is a detachment from a sense of being, remain a challenge to cognitive scientists, and are likely to involve information-processing mechanisms which are largely uncharted. How does a thought, for example, become unrecognisable as such and instead become a percept which is 'heard' by the subject? Presumably, Beck would attribute the perceived source of the percept to a dysfunctional 'self-monitoring schema', and there is much work to be done in building sound models of self-monitoring processes.

Sims (1988) feels that good practice is a balance between prior knowledge and empathy. As Sims puts it:

> Phenomenology, the empathic method for the eliciting of symptoms, can never be learned from a book. Patients are the best teachers, but it does help to know what one is looking for, the practical, clinical aspects in which the patient describes himself, his feelings and his world.
>
> (Sims 1988: 3)

Trainees often erect causal hypotheses before becoming fully acquainted with the phenomenon in question. For example, it is frequently suggested by clinical trainees during seminars that hallucinations are simply normal, emotionally-charged percepts, consisting of disturbing thoughts and vivid imagery, and that there is a continuum between hallucinations and normal perception. However, hallucinations are sometimes weak, fuzzy percepts of which the subject is only vaguely aware. Many patients describe their auditory hallucinations as barely discernible voices which babble constantly 'in the background', reflecting that the voices are occupying the periphery of awareness and are far from having vivid clarity. Conversely, patients with obsessional intrusive thoughts and imagery report them as intensely vivid and are often shocked by their 'real' quality. Yet although the obsessional patient does not always distinguish clearly between that which has occurred in imagination and that which has occurred in the outside world, there is no breakdown in contrastive analysis between percepts arising from interoceptive and exteroceptive events.

In order to overcome bias in attempts to observe and understand, Husserl advocates the suspension of contemporaneous concerns, so that the observer is detached from the business of everyday life and extricates himself from concerns peripheral to the focus of attention. Husserl is alluding to a slightly altered state of consciousness, involving intensely restricted awareness, which he terms 'aporia', or confusion, which arises when a stimulus event is studied out of context, stranded in isolation. According to Husserl, this results in a disposition of wonderment at the neutralisation of previous assumptions and at the new exposed horizon of potential possibilities of understanding. Husserl recommends the attainment of this particular frame of mind in order to be detached and devoid of observational bias. This state is similar in nature to both aesthetic experience (see Chapter 9), and *jamais vu* (see Chapter 6) in that there is emotional disinvestment in the percept attended to. Kant's notion of 'disinterest' is of relevance here and might be better renamed 'disinvested interest', in the sense that the event of interest is clearly focused on the centre of awareness, but is viewed dispassionately.

In 1901, in the first edition of the *Logical Investigations*, Husserl wrote: 'Phenomenology is descriptive psychology. . . . Pure description is a preparatory step towards theory but it is not theory itself'. But what is pure description? Spiegelberg (1975) specifically warns against rushing in and describing, since one is unlikely to suspend judgements and assumptions. When reading Husserl and Spiegelberg, it is clear that what these authors mean by description is really a highly stylised way of seeing. They talk not just of the academic excercise of putting aside historical, axiomatic and causal aspects of the object of study, but of transcendence – developing a sense of 'wonder' as psychological presentations are seen as 'meant' rather than caused. Husserl describes preliminary stages in the development of this descriptive style of seeing. For Husserl the starting point of transcendence is apperception, where the object or problem is made the focal point of attention and the horizon of attention stops with the boundaries of the object. Purity of description is not an easy task, since the observer enters the task with preconceived ideas and a preformed perceptual style, and there is a danger that these *a priori* factors will bias the observer's priorities of what is to be attended to.

Churchill (1990) suggests that phenomenological ways of seeing cannot be taught directly, but background exercises can be encouraged which will lead to better understanding of the observer's influence. Such exercises include finding out the differences between descriptive and explanatory approaches, and those between descriptive and explanatory constructs. He suggests comparing Freud and Jaspers for this purpose. According to Churchill, the student can gain a concrete sense of the difference between a descriptive language and a language of constructs that seeks to explain psychological phenomena in terms of cause and effect. He recommends exposing bias by comparing student accounts. An important step in teaching phenomenological research is confronting the student with his/her own implicit assumptions through critical reflection on the language used in describing experience. It is important for the student to realise that the data seen does not have 'stand-alone' content, but is the product of a perspective, which is inevitably perceptually biased, according to the observer's own schemata.

Some mental-health professionals find phenomenological practice difficult to digest. After all, what does one do as a phenomenologist? Unfortunately, many view phenomenology as an esoteric theoretical perspective, lacking in implications for good practice. This view can be quickly discounted when it is pointed out that whenever the patient is encouraged to give his/her account of current preoccupations, the resulting content is phenomenological data, in so far as it invariably casts light on the subjective state of the individual. Subsequent analysis remains phenomenological as long as the conclusions reached remain grounded in the personal meaning of the subject. However, clinical phenomenology is not simply about accruing masses of clinical information. There comes a point at which conclusions need to be drawn regarding a formulation of the presenting problem, which consists of a distillation of the data to hand. What the clinician initially elicits from the subject is basically a set of cognitions – attitudes, fears, preoccupations, perceptions, ways in which the subject has made sense of his or her problematic experiences. This information comprises the content of the problem, and the next important step for the clinician is to decide upon the form of these experiences, whether this represents, for example, delusional thinking, a depressive style of evaluation, alienation of thought or a disorder of self-experience. The transformation of the data from content to form requires some prior knowledge of psychopathology and adds structure to the observations that the clinician makes, without which the process would be painstakingly slow. This is particularly so of the psychoses, which may involve phenomena that the clinician finds difficult to grasp without familiarisation with phenomenological concepts. For this reason, it is recommended that students are introduced to a basic text that covers dysfunctional perception and thinking, and disorders of the sense of self. Sims (1988) is one of the most recent succinct texts on these subjects.

Experience-sampling as a research tool

An experience-sampling method developed by Dijkman and de Vries (1987) assesses rapid day-to-day and within-day fluctuations in conscious experience and its relation to mood-setting and situation. The subjects carry with them a wrist watch that signals them on a programmed random schedule. When signalled, the person completes a self-report form that includes a range of questions about his or her objective and subjective states. Reports also include information about where they are, what they are doing and who they are with as well as thoughts, moods, activities and somatic complaints. Dijkman and de Vries's results show the utility of exploring relationships between anxiety and context in revealing the social ecology of an anxiety problem. In one case, the method brought to light a number of social limitations in an anxious person's repertoire which would have gone unnoticed if a wide range of experience had not been surveyed.

Robinson (1987) advocates a 'microbehavioral' method to monitor how activities are experienced by individuals, indicating how people experience high and low points during the day. He says this represents an important advance in the clinical understanding of an individual's context and the dynamics of mood swing. Other advances on self-report techniques include 'talking aloud' procedures in which the person records their thoughts either during performance of a task, or while relating an autobiographical account. While this may be a suitable means of investigating neurotic disorders, not all patients are that co-operative while actively psychotic and others cannot be engaged in interaction when severely depressed. Nonetheless, it should not be forgotten that, when lucid, patients can provide extremely detailed retrospective accounts which give insights into the nature of their prior harrowing experiences. Some psychotic patients are uncooperative during florid episodes, or are so distracted that a dialogue is not possible at that time. This does not mean that a personal description of the experience of a florid psychosis is unobtainable. Many patients can provide detailed and thorough accounts of their psychotic state retrospectively and many of the observations of clinicians such as Schneider and Jaspers have been obtained in this way. There are shortcomings to subjective retrospective data, since experiences are often difficult to access owing to state-dependent recall, but can be matched against future observations in patients who frequently relapse. When approached in a tactful manner, and when the intentions of the clinician are made explicit, most patients, even during the florid phase of a breakdown, are able to provide a rich array of subjective information.

SUMMARY

Some of Beck's most influential contributions to the therapy literature were his ideas concerning the organisation of cognitive processes in terms of schema. Schemas are said to underlie overt features of emotions, cognitions and behaviour. Conceptually, schemas represent an attempt by the therapy fraternity to construct a psychology of covert processes to account for the maintenance of psychological disorders.

Schemata are conceptually well placed to expand information-processing research in the area of cognitive therapy. The formation and longitudinal development of schemata is an area ripe for research, though an operational definition of schemas needs to be developed in the process. The notion of Early Maladaptive Schemas will no doubt inspire much research into the aetiological status of remote events, earlier in the patient's history. Traumatic events of childhood are often systematically 'forgotten', remaining outside the recall of many patients. While psychoanalysts might regard the repression of such events as a psychoactive process precipitating lack of well-being, cognitive therapists might suggest an alternative pathogenic process: disturbing events are not simply stored as a record of the concrete experience. Perception of the event may also affect the subsequent structure and activation of latent schemas. It is the changed ways of construing, brought about by re-organisation of perception rather than memory-of-events which transmits a traumatic experience into the present experience, or 'Dasein' of the patient.

The idea that depression and paranoia are irreducible feeling states is brought into question by attributional research. The empirical observation, now replicated, that paranoid delusions are associated with a particular attributional style of regarding self in relation to external events invites the hypothesis that maladaptive attributional schemata determine whether the feeling that emerges is sadness or suspicion.

Traditional differences in emphasis have evolved between cognitive psychology and phenomenological psychiatry. While cognitive psychologists have tended to concentrate on self-concept, phenomenological psychiatrists have concentrated more on the degree to which experiences are authentic to the beholder, an area sometimes referred to as self-experience. While self-concept refers to aspects of self-image and self-schemata, self-experience refers to the degree to which thinking, imagery and other percepts are appreciated as belonging to the self. The differentiation of inner experience from distal events is a complex process which, as our hallucinating patients remind us, should not be taken for granted. When self-experience is faulty, the boundaries between self and world are eroded, and in extreme form, percepts are not felt to be internally experienced and become hallucinatory in form.

It is generally felt that phenomenological skills in the clinical setting are sharpened by prior knowledge of the various forms experience can take. Many painstaking hours of clinical observation have gone into the development of a model of psychopathology which expresses the structure of experience according to its 'lived-in' quality, since psychotic experiences often involve a perceived absence of self-participation. In depersonalisation, the loss of 'I-ness' in 'my' experiences is evaluated as a bizarre paradox, while in hallucinated individuals, aspects of conscious activity are perceived as foreign to the individual.

Though there has been a tendency for some cognitive theorists to 'explain' the occurrence of delusions in terms of attribution, their illuminating accounts are descriptive rather than explanatory. The *dasein* analysis of delusional atmosphere and delusional perception is uncharted territory for current theories of emotion. Nonetheless, the sudden shift from perplexity and guardedness to the rush of felt-meaning which patients experience during delusional perception is emotionally charged. Hopefully, theorists of emotion and cognition will explore new avenues to describe the onset of such psychotic experience.

References

Abed, R. T. and Fewtrell, W. D. (1990). 'Delusional misidentification of familiar inanimate objects'. *British Journal of Psychiatry* 157, 915–917.

Abernathy, E. M. (1940). 'The effects of changed environmental conditions upon the results of college examinations'. *Journal of Psychology* 10, 293–301.

Abernethy, B. (1988). 'Dual-task methodology and motor skills research: some applications and methodological constraints'. *Journal of Human Movement Studies* 14, 101–132.

Abse, W. (1982). 'Multiple personality'. In A. Roy (ed.) *Hysteria*. Chichester: John Wiley.

Ackner, B. (1954). 'Depersonalisation'. *Journal of Mental Science* 100, 838–872.

Afzelius, L., Mendriksson, N. G. and Waohlgren, L. (1980). 'Vertigo and dizziness of functional origin'. *The Laryngoscope* 90, 469–656.

Alford, B. A. and Beck, A. T. (1994). 'Cognitive therapy of delusional beliefs'. *Behavioural Research and Therapy* 32(3), 369–380.

Allport, G. (1943). 'The ego in contemporary psychology'. In *Personality and Social Encounter*. Boston: Beacon Press (1960).

Anderson, D. N. (1988). 'The delusion of inanimate doubles: implications for understanding the Capgras syndrome'. *British Journal of Psychiatry* 153, 694–699.

Anderson, W. (1938). 'A clinical study of states of "ecstasy" occurring in affective disorders'. *Journal of Neurological Psychiatry* 1, 1–20.

Archer, J. and Reisor, J. (1982). 'A group approach to stress and anxiety management'. *Journal for Specialists in Group Work* 7(4), 238–244.

Aristotle. 'De Coelo'. Quoted in P. Feyerabend (1985) *Against Method*. New Left Books, 58.

Asberg, M., Montgomery, S. A., Perris, C., *et al.* (1978). 'A comprehensive psychopathological rating scale'. *Acta Psychiatrica Scandinavica* (suppl. 271), 5–29.

Averill, J. R. (1975). 'A semantic atlas of emotion concepts'. *JSAS Catalog of Selected Documents in Psychology* 5, 330 (Ms. N. 421).

Averill, J. R. (1980). 'Emotions and anxiety: sociocultural, biological, and psychological determinants'. In A. Rorty (ed.) *Explaining Emotions*. Berkeley: University of California Press.

Ax, A. F. (1953). 'The physiological differentiation of fear and anger in humans'. *Psychosomatic Medicine* 15: 433–42.

Baars, B. J. (1986). *The Cognitive Revolution in Psychology*. New York: Guilford.

Baars, B. J. (1988). *A Cognitive Theory of Consciousness*. Cambridge: Cambridge University Press.

Babor, T. F., Brown, J. and Del Boca, F. K. (1990). 'Validity of self reports in applied research on addictive behaviors: fact or fiction'. *Behavioral Assessment* 12, 5–31.

Baddeley, A. D. (1986). *Working Memory*. Oxford: Oxford University Press.

Baker, T. B. and Brandon, T. M. (1990). 'Validity of self-reports in basic research'. *Behavioral Assessment* 12, 33–51.

Baldwin, M. W. (1992). 'Relational schemas and the processing of social information'. *Psychological Bulletin* 112(3), 461–484.

Baloh, R. W., Lyerty, H., Yee, R. D. and Monubia, V. (1984). 'Voluntary control of the human vestibulo-ocular reflex'. *Acta Otolaryngologica* 97, 1–6.

Bandura, A. (1977). 'Self-efficacy: towards a unifying theory of behavioral change'. *Psychological Review* 84, 191–215.

Barlow, D. H. and Craske, M. G. (1988). 'The phenomenology of panic'. In S. Rachman and J. D. Maser (eds) *Panic: Psychological Perspectives*. London: Erlbaum, pp. 11–35.

Barnard, P. J. and Teasdale, J. D. (1991). 'Interacting cognitive sub-systems: a systematic approach to cognitive-affective interaction and change'. *Cognition and Emotion* 1, 1–39.

Barr, C. C., Schulheis, L. W. and Robinson, D. A. (1976). 'Voluntary, non-visual control of the human vestibulo-ocular reflex'. *Acta Otolaryngology* (Stockholm) 81, 365.

Baumeister, R. F. (1982). 'A self-presentational view of social phenomena'. *Psychological Bulletin* 91, 3–26.

Beck, A. T. (1963). 'Thinking and depression: I. Idiosyncratic content and cognitive distortions'. *Archives of General Psychiatry* 9, 324–333.

Beck, A. T. (1971). 'Cognition, affect, and psychopathology'. *Archives of General Psychiatry* 24, 495–500.

Beck, A. T. (1976). *Cognitive Therapy and the Emotional Disorders*. New York: International Universities Press; London: Penguin.

Beck, A. T. (1988). 'Cognitive approaches to panic disorder: theory and therapy'. In S. Rachman and J. D. Maser (eds) *Panic: Psychological Perspectives*. London: Erlbaum, pp. 91–108.

Beck, A. T. and Emery, G. (1985). *Anxiety Disorders and Phobias: A Cognitive Perspective*. New York: Basic Books.

Beck, A. T., Freeman, A. and Associates (1990). *Cognitive Therapy of Personality Disorders*. New York: Guilford.

Beck, A. T., Hollon, S. D., Young, J. E., *et al.* (1985). 'Treatment of depression with cognitive therapy and amitriptyline'. *Archives of General Psychiatry* 42, 142–148.

Beck, A. T., Rush, A. J., Shaw, B. F. and Emery, G. (1979). *Cognitive Therapy of Depression*. Chichester: Wiley.

Beck, A. T. and Sokol-Kessler, L. (1986). 'The cognitive dysfunction inventory'. In S. Rachman and J. D. Maser (1988) *Panic: Psychological Perspectives*. London: Lawrence Erlbaum.

Beck, A. T., Ward, C. H., Mendelson, M., Mock, J. and Erbaugh, J. (1961). 'An inventory for measuring depression'. *Archives of General Psychiatry* 4, 561–571.

Bejerot, N. (1984). 'Addiction to pleasure: a biological and social-psychological theory of addiction'. In *Theories on Drug Abuse – Selected Contemporary Perspectives*. NIDA Research Monograph Series.

Bellak, I. and Small, I. (1978). *Emergency Psychotherapy and Brief Psychotherapy*. New York: Grune and Stratton.

Bentall, R. P., Jackson, H. F. and Pilgrim, D. (1988). 'Abandoning the concept of schizophrenia: some implications of validity arguments for psychological research into psychotic phenomena'. *British Journal of Clinical Psychology* 27, 303–324.

Bentall, R. P., Kinderman, P. and Karey, F. (1994). 'The self, attributional processes and abnormal beliefs: towards a model of persecutory delusions'. *Behaviour, Research and Therapy* 32(3), 331–334.

Bentall, R. P. and Pilgrim, D. (1993). 'Thomas Szasz, crazy talk and the myth of mental illness'. *British Journal of Medical Psychology* 66, 69–76.

Berkeley, G. (1724/1961). *A Treatise Concerning the Principles of Human Knowledge*. New York: Doubleday.

Berlyne, N. (1972). 'Confabulation'. *British Journal of Psychiatry* 120, 31–39.

Berner, P. (1991). 'Delusional atmosphere'. *British Journal of Psychiatry* 159 (suppl. 14), 88–93.

Berrios, G. E. (1985). 'Delusional parasitosis and physical disease'. *Comprehensive Psychiatry* 26, 395–403.

Berson, R. J. (1983). '"Capgras' Syndrome'. *American Journal of Psychiatry* 140, 969–978.

Beyts, J. (1987). 'Vestibular dysfunction'. In B. Dix and S. Stephens (eds) *Scott-Brown's Diseases of the Ear, Nose and Throat*. Chichester: Wiley.

Bidault, E., Luante, J. P. and Tzavaras, A. (1986). 'Prosopagnosia and the delusional misidentification syndrome'. *Bibliotheca Psychiatrica* 164, 80–91.

Binswanger, L. (1963). *Being-in-the-World*. J. Needleman (ed.). New York: Basic Books.

Birdwhistell, R. L. (1970). *Kinesics and Context*. Philadelphia: University Press.

Birtchnell, J. (1990). 'Interpersonal theory: criticism, modification, and elaboration'. *Human Relations* 43(12), 1183–1201.

Black, F. O. and Nashner, L. M. (1984). 'Vestibulo-spinal control differs in patients with reduced versus distorted function'. *Acta Otolaryngology* (suppl.) (Stockholm) 406, 110–114.

Blackburn, I. M. and Evunson, K. M. (1989). 'A content analysis of thoughts and emotions elicited from depressed patients during cognitive therapy'. *British Journal of Medical Psychology* 62, 23–33.

Bland, K. and Hallam, R. S. (1981). 'The relationship between response to graded exposure and marital satisfaction in agoraphobics'. *Behaviour, Research and Therapy* 19, 335–338.

Blascovich, J., Brennan, K., Tomaka, J., Kelsey, R. M., Hughes, P., Coad, M. L. and Adlin, R. (1992). 'Affect intensity and cardiac arousal'. *Journal of Personality and Social Psychology* 63(1), 164–174.

Bliss, R. E., Garvey, A. J., Heinhold, J. W., Hitchcock, J. (1989). 'The influence of situation and coping on relapse crisis outcomes after smoking cessation'. *Journal of Consulting and Clinical Psychology* 57(3), 443–449.

Bolton, N. (1987). 'Beyond method: phenomenology as an approach to consciousness'. *Journal of Phenomenological Psychology* 18, 49–58.

Bonn, J. A., Harrison, J. and Rees, W. L. (1973). 'Lactate infusion in the treatment of "free-floating" anxiety'. *Canadian Psychiatric Association Journal* 18, 41–46.

Bootsma, R. J. (1988). *The Timing of Rapid Interoceptive Actions*. Doctoral Dissertation. Amsterdam: Free University Press.

Borkovec, T. D. (1985). 'Worry: a potentially valuable concept'. *Behaviour Research and Therapy* 23, 481–482.

Bower, G. H. (1981). 'Mood and memory'. *American Psychologist* 36, 129–148.

Bower, G. H. and Gilligan, S. G. (1979). 'Remembering information related to one's self'. *Journal of Research in Personality* 13, 420–432.

Bower, G. H. and Gilligan, S. G. (1980). 'Emotional mood and remembering one's autobiography'. Unpublished manuscript: Stanford University.

Bower, G. H., Gilligan, S. G. and Monteiro, K. P. (1981). 'Selectivity of learning caused by affective states'. *Journal of Experimental Psychology: General* 110, 451–473.

Bower, G. H., Monteiro, K. P. and Gilligan, S. G. (1978). 'Emotional mood as a context of learning and recall'. *Journal of Verbal Learning and Verbal Behaviour* 17, 573–587.

Brandt, T. (1984). 'Visual vertigo and acrophobia'. In M. R. Dix and J. D. Hood (eds) *Vertigo*. New York: Wiley, 439–466.

Brandt, T. and Daroff, R. B. (1980). 'The multisensory physiological and pathological vertigo syndromes'. *Annals of Neurology* 7, 195–203.

Brentano, F. (1874/1973). *Psychology from an Empirical Standpoint*. London: Routledge and Kegan Paul.

Brett-Jones, J., Garety, P. A., Hemsley, R. (1987). 'Measuring delusional experiences: a method and its application'. *British Journal of Clinical Psychology* 26(4), 257–265.

Brewin, C. R. (1988). *Cognitive Foundations of Clinical Psychology*. London: Lawrence Erlbaum Associates.

Brown, R., Lichtenstein, E., McIntyre, K. O. and Harrington-Kostur, J. (1984). 'Effects of nicotine fading and relapse prevention on smoking cessation'. *Journal of Consulting and Clinical Psychology* 52(2), 307–308.

Bullen, J. G. and Hemsley, D. R. (1987). 'Schizoprenia: a failure to control the contents of consciousness?' *British Journal of Clinical Psychology* 26, 25–33.

Bullough, E. (1912). 'Psychical distance as a factor in art and aesthetic principle'. *British Journal of Psychology* 5, 87–118.

Burton, D., Sussman, S., Hansen, W. B., Johnson., C. A. and Flay, B. R. (1989). 'Image attributions and smoking intentions among seventh grade students'. *Journal of Applied Psychology* 19(8), 656–664.

Callaway, E., Halliday, R. and Naylor, H. (1992). 'Cholinergic activity and constraints on information processing'. *Biological Psychology* 33, 1–22.

Candido, C. L. and Romney, D. M. (1990). 'Attributional style in paranoid vs depressed patients'. *British Journal of Medical Psychology* 63, 355–363.

Capgras, J. and Carette, P. (1924). 'Illusions des sosies et complexe d'Oedipe'. *Annales medico-psychologiques* 82, 48–68.

Capgras, J., Lucchini, P. and Schiff, P. (1924). 'Du sentiment d'étrangeté à l'illusion des sosies'. *Bulletin de la Société Clinique de Médicine Mentale* 121, 210–217.

Capgras, J. and Reboul-Lachaux, J. (1923). 'L'illusion des sosies dans un délire systematique chronique'. *Bulletin de la Société Clinique de Médecine Mentale* 11, 6–16.

Cappon, D. and Banks, R. (1969a). 'Orientational perceptions: III. Orientational percept distortions in depersonalization'. *American Journal of Psychiatry* 125(8), 1048–1055.

Cappon, D. and Banks, R. (1969b). 'Orientational perception: IV. Time and length perception in depersonalized and derealized patients and controls under positive feedback conditions'. *American Journal of Psychiatry* 125(9), 1214–1217.

Carr, V. (1988). 'Patients' techniques for coping with schizophrenia: an exploratory study'. *British Journal of Medical Psychology* 61, 339–352.

Cawthorne, T. (1945). 'Vestibular injuries'. *Proceedings of Medicine* 39, 270.

Chambless, D. L. and Gracely, J. (1989). 'Fear of fear and the anxiety disorders'. *Cognitive Therapy and Research* 13(1), 9–20.

Charbonneau, J. and O'Connor, K. (1993). (Submitted for publication). 'Depersonalization in a non-clinical sample'.

Christodoulou, G. N. (1977). 'The syndrome of Capgras'. *British Journal of Psychiatry* 130, 564.

Christodoulou, G. N. (ed.) (1986a). 'The origin of the syndrome of doubles'. In *The Delusional Misidentification Syndromes*. Basel: Karger.

Christodoulou, G. N. (ed.) (1986b). 'Role of depersonalization-derealization phenomena in the delusional misidentification syndromes'. Basel: Karger.

Christodoulou, G. N. (1991). 'The delusional misidentification syndromes'. *British Journal of Psychiatry* 159 (suppl. 14), 65–69.

Christodoulou, G. N. and Malliara-Loulakaki, S. (1981). 'Delusional misidentification syndromes and cerebral "dysrhythmia"'. *Psychiatrica Clinica* 14, 245–51.

Churchill, S. C. (1990). 'Considerations for teaching a phenomenological research'. *Journal of Phenomenological Psychology* 21, 46–67.

Clark, D. B., Leslie, M. I. and Jacob, R. G. (1992). 'Balance complaints and panic disorder: a clinical study of panic symptoms in members of a self-help group for balance disorders'. *Journal of Anxiety Disorders* 6, 47–53.

Clark, D. M. (1986). 'Cognitive approach to panic'. *Behavior Research and Therapy* 24, 461–470.

Clark, D. M. (1988). 'A cognitive model of panic attacks'. In S. Rachman and J. D. Maser (eds) *Panic: Psychological Perspectives*. London: Erlbaum, pp. 71–87.

Cohen, A. S., Barlow, D. H. and Blanchard, E. B. (1985). 'The psychophysiology of relaxation-associated panic attacks'. *Journal of Abnormal Psychology* 94, 96–101.

Coleman, S. M. (1933). 'Misidentification and non-recognition'. *Journal of Mental Science* 79, 42–51.

Collingwood, R. G. (1938). *The Principles of Art*. Oxford: Oxford University Press.

Cooley, C. H. (1902/1956). *The two major works of Charles H. Cooley: Social Organization and Human Nature and the Social Order*. New York: Free Press.

Corty, E., Ball, J. C. and Myers, C. P. (1988). 'Psychological symptoms in methadone maintenance patients: prevalence and change over treatment'. *Journal of Consulting and Clinical Psychology* 56(5), 776–777.

Crary, W. G. and Wexler, M. (1977). 'Ménière disease: a psychosomatic disorder?' *Psychological Reports* 41, 603–645.

Crichton, P. and Lewis, S. (1990). 'Delusional misidentification, AIDS and the right hemisphere'. *British Journal of Psychiatry* 157, 608–610.

Csikszentmihalyi, M. (1974). 'Flow: studies in enjoyment'. PHS Grant Report N. RO1HM 22883-02.

Csikszentmihalyi, M. (1975). *Beyond Boredom and Anxiety*. San Francisco: Jossey-Bass.

Csikszentmihalyi, M. and Csikszentmihalyi, I. S. (1988). *Optimal Experience: Psychological Studies of Flow in Consciousness*. New York: Cambridge University Press.

Cuclos, S. E., Laird, J. D., Schneider, E., Sexter, M., Stern, L. and Van Lighten, O. (1989). 'Emotion-specific effects of facial expressions and postures on emotional experience'. *Journal of Personality and Social Psychology* 57(1), 100–108.

Curry, S. J., Marlatt, G. A., Gordon, J. and Baer, J. S. (1988). 'A comparison of alternative theoretical approaches to smoking cessation and relapse'. *Health Psychology* 7(6), 545–556.

Cutting, J. (1985). *The Psychology of Schizophrenia*. Edinburgh: Churchill Livingstone.

Cutting, J. (1991). 'Delusional misidentification and the role of the right hemisphere in the appreciation of identity'. *British Journal of Psychiatry* 159 (suppl. 14), 70–75.

Darwin, C. (1872). *Expression of Emotion in Man and Animals*. London: John Murray.

David, A. S. (1994). 'Thought echo reflects the activity of the phonological loop'. *British Journal of Clinical Psychology* 33, 81–83.

David, A. S. and Lucas, P. A. (1993). 'Auditory-verbal hallucinations and the phonological loop: a cognitive neuropsychological study'. *British Journal of Clinical Psychology* 32, 431–441.

Davison, K. (1964). 'Episodic depersonalisation: observations of seven patients.' *British Journal of Psychiatry* 110, 505–513.

Deci, E. L. and Ryan, R. M. (1985). *Intrinsic Motivation and Self-Determination in Human Behavior*. New York: Plenum Press.

De Koning, A. J. J. and Jenner, F. A. (eds) (1982). *Phenomenology and Psychiatry*. London: Academic Press.

Dennett, D. C. (1978). *Brainstorms*. Montgomery, Vermont: Bradford Books.

Denzin, N. K. (1984). *On Understanding Emotion*. San Francisco: Jossey Bass.

Descartes, R. (1644/1966). *Discourse on Method*. (Trans. Wollaston). Harmondsworth: Penguin.

Dijkman, C. I. M. and De Vries, M. W. (1987). 'The social ecology of anxiety. Theoretical and quantitative perspectives'. *The Journal of Nervous and Mental Disease* 175(19), 550–557.

Dix, M. R. and Hood, J. (eds) (1984). *Vertigo*. Chichester: John Wiley.

Dixon, J. C. (1963). 'Depersonalization phenomenon in a sample population of college students'. *British Journal of Psychiatry* 109, 371–375.

Dixon, N. F. (1971). *Subliminal Perception: The Nature of a Controversy*. London: McGraw-Hill.

Drachman, D. A. and Hart, C. M. (1972). 'An approach to the dizzy patient'. *Neurology* 22(4), 323–334.

DSM-III-R (1987). *Diagnostic and Statistical Manual* (rev. 3rd edn). Washington D.C.: American Psychiatric Press.

Dugas, I. and Moutier, F. (1911). *La Depersonalisation*. Paris: Felix Alcon.

Edelmann, R. J. (1987). *The Psychology of Embarrassment*. New York: John Wiley & Sons.

Ehlers, A., Margraf, J., Roth, W. T., Taylor, C. B. and Birbaumer, N. (1986). 'Anxiety induction by false heart rate feedback in patients with panic disorder'. Unpublished manuscript. Reported in S. Rachman and J. D. Maser (eds) *Panic: Psychological Perspectives* London: Erlbaum.

Eich, J. E. (1980). 'The cue-dependent nature of state dependent retrieval'. *Memory and Cognition* 8, 157–173.

Ekman, P. (ed.) (1982). *Emotion in the Human Face*. New York: Cambridge University Press.

Ekman, P. and Friesen, W. (1976). *Pictures of Facial Affect*. Palo Alto, California: Consulting Psychologists Press.

Ekman, P. and Oster, M. (1979). 'Facial expression of emotion'. *Annual Review of Psychology* 30, 527–554.

Elliott, R. and James, E. (1989). 'Varieties of client experience in psychotherapy: an analysis of the literature'. *Clinical Psychology Review* 9, 443–467.

Ellis, A. (1962). *Reason and Emotion in Psychotherapy*. Secausus, N.J.: Citadel.

Ellis, H. D., Young, A. W. (1990). 'Accounting for delusional misidentifications'. *British Journal of Psychiatry* 157, 239–248.

Ellis, R. J. and Zanna, M. P. (1990). 'Arousal and causal attribution'. *Canadian Journal of Behavioural Science* 22(1), 1–2.

Enoch, D. M. (1986). 'Whose Double?' In G. N. Christodolou (ed.) *The Delusional Misidentification Syndromes*. Basel: Karger.

Enoch, D. M. and Trethowan, W. (1967). 'The Capgras syndrome'. In *Some Uncommon Psychiatric Syndromes*. Bristol: John Wright and Sons.

Enoch, D. M. and Trethowan, W. (1991). *Uncommon Psychiatric Syndromes*. Oxford: Butterworth-Heinemann.

Eysenck, H. J. (1968). 'A theory of the incubation of anxiety/fear responses'. *Behaviour Research and Therapy* 6, 309–321.

Eysenck, H. J. (1980). *The Causes and Effects of Smoking*. London: Maurice Temple Smith.

Eysenck, H. J. and Eysenck, S. B. G. (1968). *Manual for the Eysenck Personality Inventory*. San Diego: Educational and Industrial Testing Service.

Fenigstein, A. and Carver, C. S. (1978). 'Self-focusing effects of heartbeat feedback'. *Journal of Personality and Social Psychology* 11, 1241–1250.

Fennell, M. J. V. and Teasdale, J. D. (1987). 'Cognitive therapy of depression: individual differences in the process of change'. *Cognitive Therapy and Research* 11, 253–272.

Ferster, C. B. and Skinner, B. F. (1957). *Schedules of Reinforcement*. New York: Appleton-Century-Crofts.

Festinger, L. (1954). 'A theory of social comparison processes'. *Human Relations* 7: 117–40.

Festinger, L. (1957). *Cognitive Dissonance*. Stanford, California: Stanford University Press.

Festinger, L., Burnham, C. A., Ono, H. and Bamber, D. (1967). 'Efference and the conscious experience of perception'. *Journal of Experimental Psychology Monograph* 74(4), 1–36.

Fewtrell, W. D. (1984). 'Relaxation and depersonalisation'. *British Journal of Psychiatry* 145, 217.

Fewtrell, W. D. (1986a). 'The problem of depersonalization in clinical practice'. Paper presented at the BPS Conference, London, 6 December.

Fewtrell, W. D. (1986b). 'Depersonalisation: a description and suggested strategies'. *British Journal of Guidance and Counselling* 34, 263–269.

Fewtrell, W. D. and O'Connor, K. P. (1988). 'Dizziness and depersonalisation'. *Advances in Behaviour and Research Therapy* 10, 201–218.

Fish, F. (1965). *Clinical Psychopathology*. M. Hamilton (ed.). Bristol: Wright.

Fish, F. (1967). *Clinical Psychopathology*. Bristol: John Wright.

Flanagan, O. J. (1992). 'The science of the mind'. In *Consciousness*. Cambridge, Mass: MIT Press.

Fonberg, E. (1986). 'Amygdala, emotions, motivation and depressive states'. In R. Plutchick and H. Kellerman (eds) *Emotion, Theory, Research and Experience*, vol. 3. London: Academic Press.

Forgas, J. P. and Bower, G. H. (1987). 'Mood effects on person-perception judgments'. *Journal of Personality and Social Psychology* 53(1), 53–60.

Fowler, D. and Morley, S. (1989). 'The cognitive-behavioural treatment of hallucinations and delusions: a preliminary study'. *Behavioural Psychotherapy* 17, 267–82.

Frank, J. D. (1986). 'Psychotherapy – the transformation of meanings: discussion paper'. *Journal of the Royal Society of Medicine* 79, 341–346.

Frank, J. D. (1987). 'Psychotherapy, rhetoric, and hermeneutics: implications for practice and research'. *Psychotherapy* 24(3), 293–302.

Frankl, V. (1952). *Logotherapy*. London: Penguin.

Frankl, V. (1957). *Psychotherapy and Existentialism*. Harmondsworth: Penguin.

Frankl, V. (1963). *Man's Search for Meaning*. New York: Washington Square.

Franks, D. D. (ed.) (1989). 'Power and role-taking: a social behaviorist's synthesis of Kemper's power and status model'. In: D. D. Franks and E. D. McCarthy (eds) *The Sociology of Emotions: Original Essays and Research Papers*. Greenwich, CT, and London: JAI Press Inc., pp. 153–178.

Franks, D. D. and McCarthy, E. D. (eds) (1989). *The Sociology of Emotions: Original Essays and Research Papers*. Greenwich, CT, and London: JAI Press Inc., pp. 51–72.

Freeman, A., Pretzer, J., Fleming, B. and Simon, K. M. (eds) (1990). *Clinical Applications of Cognitive Therapy*. New York and London: Plenum Press.

Freud, S. (1957). 'The unconscious'. In J. Strachey (ed.) *Standard Edition of the Complete Psychological Works of Sigmund Freud*, vol. 14, pp. 159–215. London: Hogarth Press. (Original work published 1915.)

Friederici, A. D. and Levelt, W. J. M. (1987). 'Resolving perceptual conflicts: the cognitive mechanism of spatial orientation'. *Aviation, Space, and Environmental Medicine* 58(9, suppl.), A164-A169.

Frijda, N. (1987). *The Emotions*. New York: Cambridge University Press.

Frith, C. D. (1971). 'Smoking behaviour and its relation to the smokers' immediate experience'. *British Journal of Social and Clinical Psychology* 10, 73–78.

Frith, C. D. (1987). 'The positive and negative symptoms of schizophrenia reflect impairments in the perception and initiation of action'. *Psychological Medicine* 17, 631–648.

Fry, R. (1937). *Vision and Design*. London: Penguin.

Galdston, I. (1947). 'On the etiology of depersonalisation'. *Journal of Nervous and Mental Diseases* 105, 25–39.

Gale, A. and Baker, S. (1981). 'In vivo or in vitro? Some effects of laboratory environments with particular reference to the psychophysiology experiment'. In M. J. Christie and P. G. Mellett (eds) *Foundations of Psychosomatics*. London: John Wiley & Sons.

Garety, P. (1985). 'Delusions: problems in definition and measurement'. *British Journal of Medical Psychology* 58, 25–34.

Garety, P., Hemsley, D. R. and Wessely, S. (1991). 'Reasoning in deluded schizophrenic and paranoid subjects: biases in performance based on a probabilistic inference task'. *Journal of Nervous and Mental Disorders* 179, 194–201.

Garfinkel, H. (1967). *Studies in Ethnomethodology*. New Jersey: Prentice-Hall.

Gendlin, E. T. (1981). *Focusing*. New York: Bantam Books.

Giorgi, A. (1992). 'Description versus interpretation: competing alternative strategies for qualitative research'. *Journal of Phenomenological Psychology* 23(2), 119–135.

Gergen, K. J. (1982). 'From self to science: what is there to know?' In J. Suls (ed) *Psychological Perspectives on Self.* Hillsdale, NJ: Lawrence Erlbaum.

Getzels, J. W. and Csikszentmihalyi, M. (1976). *The Creative Vision: A Longitudinal Study of Problem Finding in Art.* New York: Wiley Interscience.

Gibson, J. J. (1966). *The Senses Considered as Perceptual Systems.* Boston: Houghton Mifflin.

Gibson, J. J. (1979). *The Ecological Approach to Visual Perception.* Boston: Houghton Mifflin.

Gilbert, D. J. (1979). 'Paradoxical tranquilizing and emotion-reducing effects of nicotine'. *Psychological Bulletin* 86, 643–661.

Gilbert, P. (1993). 'Defence and safety: their function in social behaviour and psychopathology'. *British Journal of Clinical Psychology* 32, 131–153.

Gilligan, S. G. and Bower, G. H. (1984). 'Cognitive consequences of emotional arousal'. In E. C. Izard, J. Kagan and R. B. Zajonc (eds) *Emotions, Cognition, and Behavior.* Cambridge: Cambridge University Press.

Gilman, T. (1993). 'An investigation into the formation of delusional beliefs in the pathogenesis of Capgras syndrome'. MSc thesis (unpublished). University College, London.

Ginsberg, D., Hall, S. M. and Rosinski, M. (1992). 'Partner support, psychological treatment, and nicotine gum in smoking treatment: an incremental study'. *The International Journal of the Addictions* 27(5), 503–514.

Giorgi, A. (ed.) (1985). *Phenomenology and Psychological Research.* Pittsburgh: Duquesne Univesity Press.

Glasgow, R. E., Morray, K. and Lichtenstein, E. (1989). 'Controlled smoking versus abstinence as a treatment goal: the hopes and fears may be unfounded'. *Behavior Therapy* 20, 77–91.

Godden, D. R. and Baddeley, A. D. (1975). 'Context-dependant memory in two natural environments: on land and under water'. *British Journal of Psychology* 66, 325–331.

Goodenough, D. R. (1976). 'The role of individual differences in field dependence as a factor of learning and memory'. *Psychological Bulletin* 83(4), 675–695.

Gray, J. A. (1982). *The Neuropsychology of Anxiety.* Oxford: Oxford University Press.

Gray, J. A. (1987). *The Psychology of Fear and Stress*, 2nd edn. Cambridge: Cambridge University Press.

Green, M. F. and Kinsbourne, M. (1990). 'Subvocal activity and auditory hallucinations: clues for behavioural treatments'. *Schizophrenia Bulletin* 16, 617–625.

Greenberg, L. S. and Safran, J. D. (1987). *Emotion in Psychotherapy.* New York: Guilford Press.

Gross, J. J. and Levenson, R. W. (1993). 'Emotional suppression: physiology, self-report and expressive behavior'. *Journal of Personality and Social Psychology* 64(6), 970–986.

Guidano, V. F. (1987). *Complexity of the Self: A Developmental Approach to Psychopathology and Therapy.* New York: Guilford Press.

Guidano, V. F. (1991). 'Affective change events in a cognitive therapy system approach'. In J. D. Safran and L. S. Greenberg (eds) *Emotion, Psychotherapy, and Change.* New York and London: The Guilford Press.

Guntrip, H. (1968). *Schizoid Phenomena: Object Relations and the Self.* London: Hogarth.

Hallam, R. S. (1985). *Anxiety: Psychological Perspective on Panic and Agoraphobia.* London: Academic Press.

Hallam, R. S. and Stephens, S. D. G. (1985). 'Vestibular disorder and emotional distress'. *Journal of Psychosomatic Research* 129(4), 407–413.

Hallstrom, C. and Lader, M. (1982). 'The incidence of benzodiazepine dependence in long-term users'. *Journal of Psychiatric Treatment and Evaluation*, 4(3), 293–296.

Hampson, S. E. (1992). 'The emergence of personality: a broader context for biological perspectives'. In A. Gale and M. W. Eysenck (eds) *Handbook of Individual Differences: Biological Perspectives*. Chichester: John Wiley and Sons.

Hansen, R. D., Hansen, C. H. and Crano, W. D. (1989). 'Sympathetic arousal and self-attention: the accessibility of interoceptive and exteroceptive arousal cues'. *Journal of Experimental Social Psychology* 25, 437–449.

Harlow, H. F. (1953). 'Mice, monkeys, men, and motives'. *Psychological Review* 60, 23–32.

Harper, M. and Roth, M. (1962). 'Temporal lobe epilepsy and the phobic anxiety-depersonalisation syndrome'. *Comprehensive Psychiatry* vol. 3, 129–151.

Harré, R and Secord, P. F. (1972). *The Explanation of Social Behavior*. Oxford: Blackwell.

Havassy, B. E., Hall, S. M. and Wasserman, D. A. (1991). 'Social support and relapse: Commonalities among alcoholics, opiate users, and cigarette smokers'. *Addictive Behaviors* 16, 235–246.

Hayes, S. C. and Hayes, L. J. (1992). 'Some clinical implications of contextualistic behaviorism: the example of cognition'. *Behavior Therapy* 23, 225–249.

Hayman, M. A. and Abrams, R. (1977). 'Capgras syndrome and cerebral dysfunction'. *British Journal of Psychiatry* 130, 68–71.

Heather, N. and Bradley, B. P. (1990). 'Cue exposure as a practical treatment for addictive disorders: why are we waiting?' *Addictive Behaviors* 15, 335–337.

Hebb, D. O. (1949). *The Organization of Behavior*. New York: Wiley.

Hebb, D. O. (1955). 'Drives and the C.N.S. (Conceptual Nervous System)'. *Psychological Review* 62, 243–254.

Heckhausen, H. and Beckman, J. (1990). 'Action slips.' *Psychological Review* 97, 36–48.

Hegel, G. (1807/1929). *Die Phänomenologie des Geistes*. Hamburg: Meiner.

Hegel, G. (1931). *The Phenomenology of Mind*. London: J. Ballie, 1931.

Heide, F. J. and Borkovec, T. D. (1983). 'Relaxation-induced anxiety: paradoxical anxiety enhancement due to relaxation training'. *Journal of Consulting and Clinical Psychology* 51, 171–82.

Heidegger, M. (1927). *Being and Time*. London: SCM Press, 1962.

Heider, F. (1958). *The Psychology of Interpersonal Relations*. New York: Wiley.

Henningfield, J. E., Cohen, C. and Heishman, S. J. (1991). 'Drug self-administration methods in abuse liability evaluation'. *British Journal of Addiction* 86, 1571–1577.

Henningfield, J. E., Cohen, C. and Slade, J. D. (1991). 'Is nicotine more addictive than cocaine?' *British Journal of Addiction* 86, 565–569.

Henry, G., Weingartner, H. and Murphy, D. (1973). 'Influence of affective states and psychoactive drugs on verbal learning and memory'. *American Journal of Psychiatry* 130, 966–971.

Hibbert, G. A. (1984a). 'Hyperventilation as a cause of panic attacks'. *British Medical Journal* 288, 263–264.

Hibbert, G. A. (1984b). 'Ideational components of anxiety: their origin and content'. *British Journal of Psychiatry* 144, 618–624.

Hibbert, G. A. (1986). 'The diagnosis of hyperventilation using ambulatory carbon dioxide monitoring'. In H. Lacey and J. Stugeon (eds) *Proceedings of the 15th European Conference on Psychosomatic Medicine*.

Higgit, A., Lader, M. and Fonagy, P. (1985). 'Clinical management of benzodiazepine dependence'. *British Medical Journal* 291, 688.

Higgitt, A., Golombok, S., Fonagy, P., Lader, M. (1987). 'Group treatment of benzodiazepine dependence'. *British Journal of Addiction* 82(5), 517–523.

Hinchcliffe, R. (1967). 'Emotion as a precipitating factor in Ménière disease'. *Journal of Laryngology and Otology* 81, 471–475.

Hingley, S. M. (1992). 'Psychological theories of delusional thinking: in search of integration'. *British Journal of Medical Psychology* 65, 347–356.

Hinoki, M. (1985). 'Role of the visceral brain in body equilibrium'. *Acta OtoLaryngologia* suppl. 419, 30–52.

Hollan, S. D. and Kendall, P. C. (1980). 'Cognitive self-statements in depression: development of an Automatic Thought Questionnaire'. *Cognitive Therapy Research* 4, 383–395.

Horowitz, M. J. (ed.) (1991). *Person Schemas and Maladaptive Interpersonal Patterns*. Chicago: University of Chicago Press.

Horton, P. C., Gewirtz, M. and Hreuter, K. J. (1992). 'Alexinthyma – state and trait'. *Psychotherapy and Psychosomatics* 58, 91–96.

Hughes, J. R. and Hatsukami, D. (1986). 'Signs and symptoms of tobacco withdrawal'. *Archives of General Psychiatry* 43, 289–294.

Hughes, J. R., Higgins, S. T., Bickel, W. K., Hunt, W. K., Fenwick, J. W., Gulliver, S. B. and Mireault, G. C. (1991). 'Caffeine self-administration, withdrawal, and adverse effects among coffee drinkers'. *Archives of General Psychiatry* 48, 611–617.

Hughes, J. R., Keenan, R. M. and Yellin, A. (1989). 'Effect of tobacco withdrawal on sustained attention'. *Addictive Behaviors* 14, 577–580.

Hume, D. (1774/1961). *An Enquiry Concerning Human Understanding*. New York: Doubleday.

Husserl, E. (1967). *Ideas: General Introduction to Phenomenology* (Trans. W. R. Boyce Gibson). London: Allen and Unwin. (Originally published 1913.)

Husserl, E. (1970a). *The Crisis of European Sciences and Transcendental Phenomenology*. Evanston: Northwestern University Press. (Originally published 1954.)

Husserl, E. (1970b). *Logical Investigations* (vols. 1 and 2). New York: Humanities Press. (German originals, 1900, 1901.)

ICD10: Mental Disorders Glossary and Guide to International Classification of Diseases (1987). Geneva: World Health Organisation.

Izard, C. E. (1972). *The Face of Emotion*. New York: Appleton-Century-Crofts.

Izard, C. E. (1977). *Human Emotions*. New York: Plenum.

Izard, C. E. (1979). *Emotions in Personality and Psychopathology*. New York: Plenum.

Izard, C. E. (1991). 'Perspectives on emotions in psychotherapy'. In J. D. Safran and L. S. Greenberg (eds) *Emotion, Psychotherapy and Change*. New York: Guilford Press, pp. 281–289.

Jacob, R. G. (1988). 'Panic disorder and the vestibular system'. *Psychiatric Clinics of North America* 11, 361–374.

Jakes, S. (1987). 'Psychological aspects of disorders of hearing and balance'. In B. Dix and S. Stephens (eds) *Scott-Brown's Diseases of the Ear, Nose and Throat*. Wiley: Chichester.

Jakes, S. (1988). 'Otological symptoms and emotion: a review of the literature'. *Advances in Behavior and Research Therapy* 10, 53–103.

Jakes, S. and Beyts, J. (1985). 'Vestibular rehabilitation: preliminary results of a pilot study comparing head and neck exercises and vestibular habituation training'. Paper presented at the 6th Hallpike Symposium, Institute of Neurology, London.

Jakes, S. and Hemsley, D. R. (1986). 'Individual differences in reaction to brief exposure to unpatterned visual stimulation'. *Personality and Individual Differences* 7, 121–123.

James, P. T. (1992). 'Cognitive therapies'. In S. P. Tyrer (ed.) *Psychology, Psychiatry and Chronic Pain*. Oxford: Butterworth-Heineman, pp. 137–148.

James, W. (1890). *The Principles of Psychology*. New York: Holt. Reprinted by Harvard University Press (1983).

Janke, W. (1978). 'Behavior therapies in the treatment of drug dependence: methodological aspects and basic advantages and disadvantages'. In P. Deniker, D. Radouco-Thomas and A. Villeneuve (eds) *Neuro-Psychopharmacology*. Oxford and New York: Pergamon Press.

Jaspers, K. (ed.) (1963). *General Psychopathology* (trans. J. Hoenig and W. Hamilton). Manchester: Manchester University Press.

Johansson, C. E. and Fischman, M. W. (1989). 'The pharmacology of cocaine related to its abuse'. *Pharmacological Reviews* 41(1), 3–52.

Johansson, R. E. A. (1969). *The Psychology of Nirvana*. London: George Allen & Unwin.

Johnson, E. (1988). 'A phenomenological investigation of fear of the dark'. *Journal of Phenomenological Psychology* 19, 179–194.

Johnson, M. K. (1988). 'Reality monitoring: An experimental phenomenological approach'. *Journal of Experimental Psychology: General* 117(4), 390–394.

Kalant, O. J. and Kalant, H. (1976). 'Death in amphetamine users: causes and estimates of mortality'. In R. J. Gibbins *et al.* (eds) *Research Advances in Alcohol and Drug Problems*, vol. 3. New York: Wiley.

Kaney, S. and Bentall, R. P. (1989). 'Persecutory delusions and attributional style'. *British Journal of Medical Psychology* 62, 191–198.

Kanfer, F. M. and Phillips, J. S. (1970). *Learning Foundations of Behavior Therapy*. New York: Wiley.

Kant, I. (1790/1952). T*he Critique of Judgement* (trans. C. M. Meredith). Oxford University Press.

Kant, I. (1781/1965). 'The Critique of Pure Reason' (trans. N. K. Smith). New York: St Martin Press.

Kayan, A. (1984). 'Migraine and vertigo'. In M. R. Dix and J. D. Hood (eds) *Vertigo*. Chichester: John Wiley & Sons Ltd, pp. 249–265.

Kayan, A. and Hood, J. D. (1984). 'Neuro-otological manifestations of migraine'. *Brain* 107, 1123–1142.

Kelly, D. and Walter, C. (1968). 'The relationship between clinical diagnosis and anxiety, assessed by forearm blood flow'. *British Journal of Psychiatry*. 114, 611–626.

Kelly, G. A. (1955). *The Psychology of Personal Constructs* (2 volumes). New York: Norton.

Kelly, G. A. (1979). 'The psychotherapeutic relationship'. In B. Maher (ed.) *Clinical Psychology and Personality*. New York: R. E. Krieger, pp. 216–223.

Kenealy, P. M. (1986). 'The Velten mood induction procedure: a methodological review'. *Motivation and Emotion* 10, 315–335.

Kennedy, R. B. (1976). 'Self-induced depersonalisation syndrome'. *American Journal of Psychiatry* 133, 1326–1328.

Khantzian, E. J. (1984). 'An ego/self theory of substance dependence: a contemporary psychoanalytic perspective'. In *Theories on Drug Abuse – Selected Contemporary Perspectives*. NIDA Research Monograph Series, pp. 29–33.

Kierkegaard, S. (1844/1957). *The Concept of Dread* (trans. W. Lawrie). Princeton: Princeton University Press.

Kierkegaard, S. (1843/1954). *Either/Or*. Princeton University Press.

Kirsch, I. and Hyland, M. E. (1987). 'How thoughts affect the body: a metatheoretical framework'. *The Journal of Mind and Behavior* 8(3), 417–434.

Kirsch, I. (1985). 'Response expectancy as a determinant of experience and behavior'. *American Psychologist* 40, 1189–1202.

Klein, D. F. (1980). 'Anxiety reconceptualised'. *Comprehensive Psychiatry* 21, 411–427.

Kluger, P. N. and Turvey, M. T. (1987). *Information, Natural Law, and the Self-Assembly of Rhythmic Movement*. Hillsdale, NJ: Lawrence Erlbaum.

Knott, V. (1985). 'Tobacco effects on cortical evoked potentials to distracting stimuli'. *Neuropsychobiology* 13, 74–80.

Kovacs, M. and Beck, A. T. (1978). 'Maladaptive cognitive structures in depression'. *American Journal of Psychiatry* 135(5), 525–533.

Kozlowski, L. T. and Heatherton, T. F. (1990). 'Self-report issues in cigarette smoking: state of the art and future directions'. *Behavioral Assessment* 12, 53–75.

Kuiken, D., Schopflocher, D. and Wild, T. C. (1989). 'Numerically aided methods in phenomenology: a demonstration'. *The Journal of Mind and Behavior* 10(4), 373–392.

Kuiken, D. and Wild, T. C. (1988). 'Meaning horizon, paraphrase, and phenomenological investigations in psychology'. In W. J. Baker, L. P. Mos and H. Stam (eds) *Recent Trends in Theoretical Psychology*. New York: Springer-Verlag, pp. 189–198.

Kumari, N. and Blackburn, I. M. (1992). 'How specific are negative automatic thoughts to a depressed population? An exploratory study'. *British Journal of Medical Psychology* 65(2), 167–176.

Kusyszyn, I. (1990). 'Existence, effectance, esteem: from gambling to a new theory of human motivation'. *The International Journal of the Addictions* 25(2), 159–177.

Lacey, J. P. (1950). 'Individual differences in somatic response patterns'. *Journal of Comparative and Physiological Psychology* 43, 338–350.

Lacey, J. P. and Lacey, B. (1958). 'Verification and extension of the principle of autonomic response-stereotypy'. *American Journal of Psychology* 71, 50–73.

Lader, M. H. (1972). 'Psychophysiological research and psychosomatic medecine'. In *Physiology, Emotion and Psychosomatic Illness*. CIBA foundation symposium 8. Amsterdam: North Holland Elsevier, pp. 29–30.

Lader, M. H. and Wing, L. (1966). *Physiological Measures, Sedative Drugs and Morbid Anxiety*. Maudsley Monograph No. 14. London: Oxford University Press.

Laing, R. D. (1965). *The Divided Self*. Harmondsworth: Penguin.

Laird, J. D. (1974). 'Self-attribution of emotion: the effects of expressive behavior on the quality of emotional experience'. *Journal of Personality and Social Psychology* 33, 475–486.

Laird, J. D., Wagener, J. J., Halal, M. and Szegda, M. (1982). 'Remembering what you feel: the effects of emotion on memory'. *Journal of Personality and Social Psychology* 42, 646–657.

Lambert, M. J. (1989). 'The individual therapist's contribution to psychotherapy process and outcome'. *Clinical Psychology Review* 9, 469–485.

Laming, D. (1985). 'Some principles of sensory analysis'. *Psychological Review* 92(4), 462–483.

Lang, P. J. (1979a). 'A bio-informational model of processing psychophysiology'. *Psychophysiology* 11, 125–146.

Lang, P. J. (1979b). 'A bio-informational theory of emotional imagery'. *Psychophysiology* 16, 495–512.

Langer, E. (1992). 'Matter of mind: mindfulness/mindlessness in perspective'. *Consciousness and Cognition* 1, 289–305.

Latané, B. and Darley, J. M. (1970). *The Unresponsive Bystander: Why Doesn't He Help?* New York: Appleton-Century-Crafts.

Layden, M. A., Newman, C. F., Freeman, A. and Morse, S. B. (1993). *Cognitive Therapy of Borderline Personality Disorders*. New York: Allyn & Bacon.

Lazarus, R. S. (1982). 'Thoughts on the relations between emotion and cognition'. *American Psychologist* 37, 1019–1024.

Lazarus, R. S. (1984a). 'On the primacy of cognition'. *American Psychologist* 39, 124–129.

Lazarus, R. S. (1984b). 'Thoughts on the relation between emotion and cognition'. In K. S. Scherer and P. Ekman (eds) *Approaches to Emotion*. Hillsdale, NJ: Lawrence Erlbaum, pp. 247–257.

Lazarus, R. S. (1991). 'Emotion theory and psychotherapy'. In J. D. Safran and L. S. Greenberg (eds) *Emotion, Psychotherapy and Change*. New York and London: Guilford Press.

Lee, C. (1992). 'On cognitive theories and causation in human behavior'. *Journal Therapy and Experimental Psychiatry* 23(4), 251–268.

Leigh, B. C. (1989). 'Attitudes and expectancies as predictors of drinking habits: a comparison of three scales'. *Journal of Studies on Alcohol* 50(5), 432–440.

de Leon, J., Bott, A. and Simpson, G. M. (1989). 'Dysmorphophobia: body dysmorphic disorder or delusional disorder, somatic subtype?' *Comprehensive Psychiatry* 30(6), 457–472.

Lepper, M. R. and Greene, D. (eds) (1978). *The Hidden Costs of Reward: New Perspectives on the Psychology of Human Motivation*. Hillsdale, NJ: Lawrence Erlbaum.

Lesser, I. M. (1985). 'Current concepts in psychiatry: alexithymia'. *New England Journal of Medicine* 312, 690–692.

Levenson, R. W., Eckman, P. and Friesen, W. V. (1990). 'Voluntary facial action generates emotion-specific autonomic nervous activity'. *Psychophysiology* 27(4), 363–384.

Lewis, A. (1967). *The State of Psychiatry*. London: Routledge and Kegan Paul.

Lewis, N. D. C. (1949). 'Criteria for early differentiation of psychoneurosis and schizophrenia'. *American Journal of Psychotherapy* 3, 4–18.

Lewis, S. W. (1987). 'Brain imaging in a case of Capgras 'syndrome''. *British Journal of Psychiatry* 150, 117–121.

Lindenfield, G. (1992). *The Positive Woman*. London: Thorsons.

Lindesmith, A. R. (1984). 'A general theory of addiction to opiate-type drugs'. In *Theories on Drug Abuse – Selected Contemporary Perspectives*. NIDA Research Monograph Series, pp. 34–37.

Lipkin, B. (1988). 'Capgras syndrome heralding the development of dementia'. *British Journal of Psychiatry* 153, 117–118.

Locke, J. (1690/1961). *An Essay Concerning Human Understanding*. New York: Doubleday.

Loeb, L. (1981). *From Descartes to Hume*. Ithaca and London: Cornell University Press.

Ludwig, A. M. and Wikler, A. (1974) '"Craving" and relapse to drink'. *Quarterly Journal of Studies on Alcohol* 35, 108–130.

Lusebrink, V. B. (1992). 'A systems oriented approach to the expressive therapies: the expressive therapies continuum'. *The Arts in Psychotherapy* 18, 395–403.

Lyons, W. (1980). *Emotion*. Cambridge: Cambridge University Press.

McCarthy, E. D. (1989). 'Emotions are social things: an essay in the sociology of emotions'. In D. D. Franks and E. D. McCarthy (eds) *The Sociology of Emotions: Original Essays and Research Papers*. Greenwich, CT, and London: JAI Press Inc., pp. 51–72.

McGuigan, F. J. (1978). *Cognitive Psychophysiology: Principles of Covert Behavior*. Englewood Cliffs, NJ: Prentice-Hall Inc.

McGuire, F. L. (1972). 'Smoking, driver education and other correlates of accident among young males'. *Journal of Safety Research* 4, 5–11.

McGuire, W. J. (1968). 'Personality and susceptibility to social influence'. In E. F. Borgata and W. W. Lambert (eds) *Handbook of Personality Theory and Research*. Chicago: Rand McNally, pp. 1130–1187.

Mackay, P. W. and Marlatt, G. A. (1990–91). 'Maintaining sobriety: stopping is starting'. *The International Journal of the Addictions* 25(9A and 10A), 1257–1276.

McKenna, L. and O'Connor, K. P. (1987). 'A psychological approach to the rehabilitation of patients with vertigo'. Reported by L. McKenna at 8th Hallpike Symposium, London.

MacNab, B., Nieuwenhuijse, B., Jansweyer, W. and Kuiper, A. (1978). 'Height and distance ratio as a predictor of perceived openness-enclosure of space and emotional responses in normal and phobic subjects'. *Netherlands Journal of Psychology* 33, 375–388.

Macquarrie, J. (1972). *Existentialism*. Harmondsworth: Penguin.

Magnusson, P., Nilsson, A. and Mendriksson, N. (1977). 'Psychogenic vertigo within an anxiety frame of reference: an experimental study'. *British Journal of Medical Psychology* 50, 187–201.

Mahoney, M. J. (1988). 'Constructive metatheory: 1. Basic features and historical foundations'. *International Journal of Personal Construct Psychology* 1, 1–35.

Mahoney, M. J. (1991). Founder's address. World Congress of Cognitive Therapy, Toronto, Ontario.

Mahoney, M. J. and Lyddon, W. J. (1988). 'Recent developments in cognitive approaches to counselling and psychotherapy'. *The Counselling Psychologist* 16(2), 190–234.

Manding, J. J. (1982). 'Psychiatric aspects of dizziness and vertigo'. In A. J. Finestone (ed.), *Evaluation and Clinical Management of Dizziness and Vertigo*. Bristol: Wright.

Mandler, G. (1984). *Mind and Body: Psychology of Emotion and Stress*. New York: Norton.

Marks, I. (1969). *Fear and Phobias*. London: Heinemann.

Marks, I. (1981). 'Pace "phobia": a pseudo-agoraphobic syndrome'. *Journal of Neurology, Neurosurgery and Psychiatry* 44, 387–391.

Marlatt, G. A. (1985). 'Relapse prevention: theoretical rationale and overview of the model'. In G. A. Marlatt and J. R. Gordon (eds) *Relapse Prevention: Maintenance Strategies in the Treatment of Addictive Behaviors*. New York: Guilford Press, pp. 2–70.

Marlatt, G. A. and Gordon, J. R. (eds) (1985). *Relapse Prevention: Maintenance Strategies in the Treatment of Addictive Behaviors*. New York: Guilford Press, pp. 410–452.

Marsh, A. (1984). 'Smoking: habit or choice?' *Population Trends* 37, 14–20.

Marx, K. (1867/1967). *Das Kapital*. London: Penguin.

Marx, K. (1956). *Karl Marx: Selected Writings in Sociology and Social Philosophy*. T. B. Bottmore and Maximilien Rubel (eds). London: Watts.

Maslow, A. H. (1968). *Toward a Psychology of Being*. Princeton: Van Nostrand.

Mathews, A. and MacLeod, C. (1985). 'Selective processing of threat cues in anxiety states'. *Behaviour Research and Therapy* 23, 563–569.

Mathews, A. and Macleod, C. (1986). 'Discrimination of threat cues without awareness in anxiety states'. *Journal of Abnormal Psychology* 95, 131–138.

Mayer, J. D., Gaschke, Y. V., Braverman, D. L. and Evans TW (1992). 'Mood-congruent judgment is a general effect'. *Journal of Personality and Social Psychology* 63(1), 119–132.

Mayer-Gross, W. (1935). 'On depersonalisation'. *British Journal of Medical Psychology* 15, 103–122.

Mayer-Gross, W., Salter, E. and Roth, M. (1969). *Clinical Psychiatry*. London, Baillière, Tindall and Cassell.

Mead, G. H. (1934). *Mind, Self, Society*. Chicago: University of Chicago Press.

Meadows, J. C. (1974). 'The anatomical basis of prosopagnosia'. *Journal of Neurology, Neurosurgery, and Psychiatry* 37, 489–501.

Mechanic, D. (1979). 'The stability of health and illness behavior: results from 16-year follow-up'. *American Journal of Public Health* 69, 1142–1145.

Mellor, C. S. (1991). 'Delusional perception'. *British Journal of Psychiatry* 159 (suppl. 14), 104–107.

Melzack, R. (1989). 'Phantom limbs, the self and the brain'. *Canadian Psychology* 30, 1–16.

Merleau-Ponty, M. (1964). *The Primacy of Perception* (ed. J. M. Edie, trans. W. Cobb and others). Evanston, IL: Northwestern University Press.

Merleau-Ponty, M. (1965). *The Structure of Behaviour*. London: Methuen and Co.

Merleau-Ponty, M. (1968). *The Visible and the Invisible*. (C. Lefort ed. A. Lingis trans.). Evanston, IL: Northwestern University Press.

Meyer, J. E. (1956). 'Studien zur Depersonalisation'. *Psychiat. et Neurol. Basel* 132, 221–32.

Miller, G. A. (1956). 'The magical number seven, plus or minus two: some limits on our capacity for processing information'. *Psychological Review* 63, 81–97.

Miller, N. S. and Gold, M. S. (1990). 'Benzodiazepines: tolerance, dependence, abuse, and addiction'. *Journal of Psychoactive Drugs* 22(1), 23–33.

Minneker-Hügel, M., Unland, H. and Buchkremer, G. (1992). 'Behavioral relapse prevention strategies in smoking cessation'. *The International Journal of the Addictions* 27(5), 627–634.

Mischel, T. (ed.) (1977). 'Conceptual issues in the psychology of the self: an introduction'. In *The Self: Psychological and Philosophical Issues*. Totowa, NJ: Rowman and Littlefield, pp. 3–28.

Monteiro, K. P. and Bower, G. H. (1980). Data reported in Bower and Gilligan (1980) 'Emotional mood and remembering one's autobiography'. Unpublished manuscript, Stanford University.

Moran, C. (1986). 'Depersonalisation associated with marijuana use'. *British Journal of Medical Psychology* 59, 187–196.

Morris, D., Collet, P., March, P. and O'Shaughnessey, M. (1979). *Gestures*. London: Jonathan Cape.

Morris, L. (1979). *Extraversion and Introversion*. New York: Wiley.

Murphy, S. M. and Tyrer, P. (1991). 'A double-blind comparison of the effects of gradual withdrawal of lorazepam, diazepam and bromazepam in benzodiazepine dependence'. *British Journal of Psychiatry* 158, 511–516.

Murphy, S. T. and Zajonc, R. B. (1993). 'Affect, cognition and awareness: affective priming with optimal and suboptimal stimulus exposure'. *Journal of Personality and Social Psychology* 64(5), 723–739.

Nagel, T. (1974). 'What is it like to be a bat?' *Philosophical Review* 83, 435–450.

Natsoulas, T. (1992). 'Intentionality, consciousness and subjectivity'. *Journal of Mind and Behavior* 13(3), 281–308.

Neiss, R. (1988). 'Reconceptualizing arousal: psychobiological states in motor performance'. *Psychological Bulletin* 103(3), 345–366.

Neisser, U. N. (1976). *Cognition and Reality: Principles and Implications of Cognitive Psychology*. San Francisco: W. H. Freeman and Company.

Nemiah, J. C., Freyberger, M. and Sifneos, P. (1976). 'Alexthymia: a view of the psychosomatic process'. In O. W. Hill (ed.) *Modern Trends in Psychosomatic Medicine*. New York: Appleton-Century-Crofts.

Nisbett, R. E. and DeCamp Wilson, T. (1977). 'Telling more than we can know: verbal reports on mental processes'. *Psychological Review* 84(3), 231–259.

Noble, W. (1986). 'Hearing, hearing impairment and the audible world. A theoretical essay.' *British Journal of Audiology* 20, 86–95.

Norton, G. R., Dorward, J. and Cox, B. J. (1986). 'Factors associated with panic attacks in nonclinical subjects'. *Behavior Therapy* 17, 239–252.

Noyes, R. and Kletti, R. (1976). 'Depersonalisation in the face of life-threatening danger'. *Omega* 7, 103–114.

Oatley, K. and Johnson-Laird, P. N. (1987). 'Towards a cognitive theory of emotions'. *Cognition and Emotion* 1, 29–50.

Obrist, P. A. (1981). *Cardiovascular Psychophysiology: A Perspective*. New York: Plenum Press.

O'Connor, K. P. (1985). 'A model of situational preference among smokers'. *Personality and Individual Differences* 6, 151–160.

O'Connor, K. P. (1986). 'Psychological aspects of dizziness'. Proceedings of B.P.S. Conference, London, 14–15 December.

O'Connor, K. P. (1989a). 'Individual differences and motor systems in smoking behaviour'. In T. Ney and A. Gale (eds) *Smoking and Human Behaviour*. Chichester: Wiley.

O'Connor, K. P. (1989b). 'Smoking reduction based on a situational model of craving'. *Psychological Reports* 65, 963–966.

O'Connor, K. P. (1992). 'Design and analysis in individual difference research'. In A. Gale and M. W. Eysenck (eds) *Handbook of Individual Differences: Biological Perspectives*. John Wiley & Sons Ltd, pp. 45–79.

O'Connor, K. P. (1993). 'Smoking, heart rate and personality'. *Personality and Individual Differences* 14(1), 225–232.

O'Connor, K. P. and Bradley, B. (1990). 'Cognitive cues for use in a case of amphetamine sulphate abuse'. Journal of Nervous and Mental Disease 178, 4.

O'Connor, K. P., Chambers, C. and Hinchcliffe, R. (1989). 'Dizziness and perceptual style'. *Psychotherapy and Psychosomatics* 51(4), 169–174.

O'Connor, K. P., Hallam, R. S., Betys, J. and Hinchcliffe, R. (1988). 'Dizziness: behavioural, subjective and organic aspects'. *Journal of Psychosomatic Research* 32, 291–302.

O'Connor, K. P., Hallam, R. S. and Rachman, S. (1985). 'Fearlessness and courage: a replication'. *British Journal of Psychology* 76, 187–197.

O'Connor, K. P. and Langlois, R. (1991). 'Profiles of craving among smokers: smoking types or smoker types'. *Personality and Individual Differences* 12(2), 189–193.

O'Connor, K. P. and Langlois, R. (1993). 'Situational typing and graded smoking reduction'. *Psychological Reports* 72, 747–751.

O'Connor, K. P. and Physant-Skov, M. (1989). 'Smoking reduction based on a situational model of craving'. *Psychological Reports* 65, 963–966.

O'Connor, K. P. and Stravynski, A. (1982). 'Evaluation of a smoking typology by use of a specific behavioural substitution method of self-control'. *Behavioral and Research Therapy* 20, 279–288.

O'Gorman, J. G. (1973). 'Change in stimulus conditions and the orienting response'. *Psychophysiology* 10, 465–470.

Ortony, A., Clore, G. L. and Collins, A. (1988). *The Cognitive Structure of Emotions*. Cambridge: Cambridge University Press.

Osgood, C. E., Suci, G. J. and Tannenbaum, P. M. (1971). *The Measurement of Meaning*. Urbana: University of Illinois Press.

Ottaviani, R. and Best, A. T. (1987). 'Cognitive aspects of panic disorders'. *Journal of Anxiety Disorders* 1, 15–28.

Ottenbacher, K., Abbott, C., Haley, D. and Watson, P. J. (1984). 'Human figure drawing ability and vestibular processing dysfunction in learning disabled children.' *Journal of Clinical Psychology* 40(4), 1084–1089.

Overstall, P. W. (1983). 'Rehabilitation of elderly patients with disorders of balance'. In R. Minchcliffe (ed.) *Meaning and Balance in the Elderly*. Edinburgh: Churchill Livingstone.

Owen, N. and Brown, S. L. (1991). 'Smokers unlikely to quit'. *Journal of Behavioral Medicine* 14(6), 627–636.

Oxman, T. E., Rosenberg, S. D., Schnurr, P. P., Tucker, G. J. and Gala, G. (1988). 'The language of altered states'. *Journal of Nervous and Mental Disease* 176(7), 401–408.

Parker, E. S., Birnbaum, I. M. and Noble, E. P. (1976). 'Alcohol and memory: storage and state-dependancy'. *Journal of Verbal Learning and Verbal Behaviour* 15, 691–702.

Peele, S. (1984). 'Addiction to an experience: a social psychological-pharmacological theory of addiction'. In *Theories of Drug Abuse. Selected Contemporary Perspectives*. NIDA research monograph series.

Peele, S. (1985). *The Meaning of Addiction. Compulsive Experience and its Interpretation*. Lexington, MA: Lexington Books.

Peterson, C. and Seligman, M. (1984). 'Causal explanations as a risk factor for depression. Theory and evidence'. *Psychological Review* 91, 347–374.

Peterson, C., Semmel, A., von Baeyer, C., Abramson, L. Y., Metalsky, G. T. and Seligman, M. (1982). 'Attributional Style Questionnaire'. *Cognitive Therapy and Research* 6, 27–37.

Phelps, S. and Austin, N. (1987). *The Assertive Woman*. Horsham: Arlington Books.

Plutchick, R. (1962). *The Emotions: Facts, Theories, and a New Model*. New York: Random House.

Plutchick, R. (1980). 'A general psychoevolutionary theory of emotion'. In R. Plutchick and H, Kellerman (eds) *Emotion: Theory, Research and Experience*, vol. 1, pp. 3–31. New York: Academic Press.

Pole, D. (1983). *Aesthetics, Form and Emotion*. London: Duckworth.

Pomerleau, O. F. and Pomerleau, C. S. (1988). 'A biobehavioral view of substance abuse and addiction'. *Journal of Drug Issues* 17, 111–131.

Powell, J., Gray, J. A., Bradley, B. P., Kasvikis, Y., Strang, J., Barratt, L. and Marks, I. (1990). 'The effects of exposure to drug-related cues in detoxified opiate addicts: a theoretical review and some new data'. *Addictive Behaviors* 15, 339–354.

Pratt, R. T. C. and McKenzie, W. (1958). 'Anxiety states following vestibular disorders'. *The Lancet* 2, 347–349.

Quinney, R. (1988). 'Beyond the interpretive: the way of awareness'. *Sociological Inquiry* 58(1), 102–116.

Rachman, S., Levitt, K. and Lopatka, C. (1987). 'A single method of distinguishing between expected and unexpected panics'. *Behaviour Research and Therapy* 25, 149–154.

Rachman, S. and Maser, J. D. (1988). *Panic: Psychological Perspectives*. London: Erlbaum.

Rader, M. and Jessup, B. (1976). *Art and Human Values*. New Jersey: Prentice Hall, pp. 46–54.

Rallo, J. (1972). 'Aggressiveness, feeling of giddiness and muscular tension'. *International Journal of Psycho-Analysis* 53, 265–269.

Rapee, R. M. (1985). 'Distinctions between panic disorder and generalized anxiety disorder'. *Australian & New Zealand Journal of Psychiatry* 19, 227–232.

Rapee, R. M. (1986). 'Differential response to hyperventilation in panic disorder and generalized anxiety disorders'. *Journal of Abnormal Psychology* 95, 24–28.

Rapee, R. M. (1991). 'Generalized anxiety disorder: a review of clinical features and theoretical concepts'. *Clinical Psychology Review* 11, 419–440.

Rapee, R. M., Mattick, R. and Murrell, E. (1986). 'Cognitive mediation in the affective component of spontaneous panic attacks'. *Journal of Behavior Therapy & Experimental Psychiatry* 17, 245–253.

Resnick, R. B. and Resnick, E. B. (1984). 'Cocaine abuse and its treatment'. *Psychiatric Clinics of North America* 7(4), 713–728.

Rice, L. N. and Greenberg, L. S. (eds) (1984). *Patterns of Change. Intensive Analysis of Psychotherapy Process*. New York and London: The Guilford Press.

Riskind, J. H. (1983). 'Nonverbal expressions and the accessibility of life experience memories: a congruency hypothesis'. *Social Cognition* 2, 62–86.

Rizzo, A. A., Stamps, L. E. and Fehr, L. A. (1988). 'Effects of caffeine withdrawal on motor performance and heart rate changes'. *International Journal of Psychophysiology* 6, 9–14.

Roberts, W. W. (1960). 'Normal and abnormal depersonalisation'. *Journal of Mental Science* 106, 478–493.

Robins, L. N. (1984). 'The natural history of drug abuse'. In *Theories on Drug Abuse – Selected Contemporary Perspectives*. NIDA Research Monograph Series, pp. 215–224.

Robinson, J. P. (1987). 'Microbehavioral approaches to monitoring human experience'. *The Journal of Nervous and Mental Disease* 175(9), 514–518.

Rogers, C. R. (1951). *Client-Centered Therapy: Its Current Practice, Implications, and Theory*. Boston: Houghton Mifflin.

Rogers, C. R. (1961). *On Becoming a Person*. Boston: Houghton Mifflin.

Rosenfeld, H. (1947). 'Analysis of schizophrenic state with depersonalisation'. *International Journal of Psycho-Analysis* 28, 130–139.

Roth, M. (1960). 'The phobic anxiety-depersonalisation syndrome and some general aetiological problems in psychiatry'. *Journal of Neuropsychiatry* 1, 292–306.

Rotter, J. B. (1966). 'Generalised expectancies for internal versus external control of reinforcement'. *Psychological Monographs* 80(1), no. 609, pp. 1–28.

Rudge, P. and Chambers, B. R. (1982). 'Physiological basis for enduring vestibular symptoms'. *Journal of Neurology, Neurosurgery and Psychiatry* 45, 908–1004.

Safran, J. D. and Greenberg, L. S. (eds) (1991). *Emotion, Psychotherapy, and Change*. New York and London: The Guilford Press.

Safran, J. D. (1990). 'Towards a refinement of cognitive therapy in light of interpersonal theory. I. Theory, II. Practice'. *Clinical Psychology Review* 10, 87–121.

Salkovskis, P. (1985). 'Obsessional-compulsive problems. A cognitive-behavioral analysis'. *Behavior Research and Therapy* 25, 571–583.

Salkovskis, P. M. (1988). 'Phenomenology, assessment, and therapy'. In S. Rachman and J. D. Maser (eds) *Panic: Psychological Perspectives*. London: Erlbaum, pp. 112–131.

Sarbin, T. (1986). 'Emotion and act: roles and rhetoric'. In R. Harré (ed.) *Social Construction of Emotion*. Oxford: Blackwell.

Sartre, J. P. (1943/57). *Being and Nothingness*. London: Methuen.

Schachter, S. and Singer, J. E. (1962). 'Cognitive, social, and physiological determinants of emotional state'. *Psychological Review* 69, 379–399.

Scharfetter, C. (1980). *General Psychopathology: An Introduction*. Cambridge: Cambridge University Press.

Scherer, K. R. (1984). 'On the nature and function of emotion: A component approach'. In K. R. Scherer and P. Ekman (eds) *Approaches to Emotion*. Hillsdale, NJ: Erlbaum, pp. 293–318.

Scherer, K. R. (1988). 'Criteria for emotion-antecedent appraisal: a review'. In V. Hamilton, G. H. Bower and Frijda, N. H. (eds) *Cognitive Perspectives on Emotion and Motivation*. Ordrecht: Nijhoff, pp. 89–126.

Schilder, P. (1933). 'The vestibular apparatus in neurosis and psychosis'. *Journal of Nervous and Mental Diseases* 78, 137–164.

Schneider, K. (1959). *Clinical Psychopathology*, 5th edn. (trans. M. W. Hamilton). New York: Grune & Stratton.

Schraberg, M. D. and Weitzel, W. D. (1979). 'Prosopagnosia and the Capgras syndrome'. *Journal of Clinical Psychiatry* 40, 313–316.

Schultz, J. H. and Luthe, W. (1969). *Autogenic Training: A Psychophysiological Approach to Psychotherapy*. New York and London: Grune & Stratton.

Schwanenberg, E. (1990). 'The world of probability and the world of meaning: cognition and affect in perspective'. *Social Science Information* 29(2), 249–270.

Sedman, G. (1970). 'Theories of depersonalisation: a re-appraisal'. *British Journal of Psychiatry* 117, 1–14.

Seligman, M. E. P. (1975). *Helplessness: On Depression, Development, and Death*. San Francisco: Freeman.

Shean, D., Bergman, E., Hill, K., Abel, A. and Hinds, L. (1992). 'Blushing as a function of audience size'. *Psychophysiology* 29(4), 431–436.

Sherrington, C. S. (ed.) (1900). *A Textbook of Physiology*. Edinburgh and London: Pentland.

Shields, S. A. and Simon, A. (1991). 'Is awareness of bodily change in emotion related to awareness of other bodily processes?' *Journal of Personality Assessment* 57(1), 96–109.

Shiffman, S. (1979). 'The tobacco withdrawal syndrome'. In N. W. Krasnegor (ed.) *Cigarette Smoking as a Dependence Process*. Washington, DC: National Institute on Drug Abuse, pp. 158–184.

Shiffman, S. (1982). 'Relapse following smoking cessation'. *Journal of Consulting and Clinical Psychology* 50, 71–86.

Shoham-Salomon, V. (1990). 'Interrelating research processes of process research'. *Journal of Consulting and Clinical Psychology* 58(3), 295–303.

Shoham-Salomon, V., Avner, R. and Neeman, R. (1989). 'You're changed if you do and changed if you don't: mechanisms underlying paradoxical interventions'. *Journal of Consulting and Clinical Psychology* 57(5), 590–598.

Shorvon, H. J. (1946). 'The depersonalisation syndrome'. *Proceedings of the Royal Society of Medicine* 39, 779–785.

Siegel, S. (1983). 'Classical conditioning, drug tolerance, and drug dependence'. In Y. Israel, F. B. Glaser, H. Kalant, R. E. Popham, W. Schmidt and R. G. Smart (eds) *Research Advances in Alcohol and Drug Problems*. New York: Plenum Press, pp. 207–246.

Siegel, S., Krank, M. D. and Hinson, R. E. (1988). 'Anticipation of pharmacological and nonpharmacological events: classical conditioning and addictive behavior'. In S. Peele (ed.) *Visions of Addiction*. Lexington, MA: Lexington Books.

Sifneos, P. E. (1972). *Short Term Psychotherapy and Emotional Crises*. Harvard University Press.

Sims, A. C. P. (1986). 'The psychopathology of schizophrenia with special reference to delusional misidentification'. In G. M. Christodoulou (ed.) *The Delusional Misidentification Syndromes*. Basel: Karger.

Sims, A. (1988). *Symptoms in the Mind*. London: Ballière Tindall.

Skelton-Roberts, M. (1975). 'Depersonalisation'. Ph. D. thesis, University of Dundee.

Slater, E. and Roth, M. (1969). *Clinical Psychiatry*, 3rd edn. London: Baillière Tindall and Cassell.

Snaith, R. P. (1981). *Clinical Neurosis*. Oxford: Oxford University Press.

Snaith, R. P. and Taylor, C. M. (1985). 'Irritability: definition, assessment and associated factors'. *British Journal of Psychiatry* 147, 127–36.

Solomon, R. L. and Corbit, J. D. (1973). 'An opponent-process theory of motivation: II. Cigarette addiction'. *Journal of Abnormal Psychology*.

Sperry, R. W. (1991). 'In defense of mentalism and emergent interaction'. *The Journal of Mind and Behavior* 12(2), 221–246.

Sperry, R. W. (1992). 'Turnabout on consciousness: a mentalist view'. *Journal of Mind and Behavior* 13(3), 259–280.

Sperry, R. W. (1993). 'The cognitive revolution: a new paradigm for causation'. *International Journal of Psychiatry* 3(1), 3–6.

Spiegelberg, H. (1972). *Phenomenology in Psychology and Psychiatry*. Evanston: Northwestern University Press.

Spiegelberg, H. (1975). *Doing Phenomenology: Essays on and in Phenomenology*. The Hague: Martinus Nijhoff.

Spinelli, E. (1989). *The Interpreted World. An Interpreted World. An Introduction to Phenomenological Psychology*. London: Sage.

Staats, A. W. and Eifert, G. H. (1990). 'The paradigmatic behaviorism theory of emotions: Basis for unification'. *Clinical Psychology Review* 10, 539–566.

Stein, H. F. (1990). 'In what systems do alcohol/chemical addictions make sense? Clinical ideologies and practices as cultural metaphors'. *Social Science and Medicine* 30(9), 987–1000.

Stein, N. L. and Oatley, K. (1992). 'Basic emotions: theory and measurement'. *Cognition and Emotion* 6(3/4), 161–168.

Stein, N. L. and Trabasso, T. (1992). 'The organization of emotional experience: creating links among emotion, thinking and intentional action'. *Cognition and Emotion* 6(3/4), 225–244; 82, 158–171.

Stephens, S. D. G. (1975). 'Personality tests in Ménière disorder'. *Journal of Laryngology and Otology* 89, 479–490.

Stephens, S. D. G., Hogan, S. and Meredith, R. (1991). 'The desynchrony between complaints and signs of vestibular disorders'. *Acta Otolaryngoly* (Stockholm) III: (suppl. 476), 77–85.

Stevens, S. S. (1961). 'Is there a quantal threshold?' In W. A. Rosenblith (ed.) *Sensory Communication*. Boston: MIT Press.

Stewart, W. F., Linet, M. S. and Celentano, D. D. (1989). 'Migraine headaches and panic attacks'. *Psychosomatic Medicine* 51, 559–569.

Stitzer, M. L. and Gross, J. (1988). 'Smoking relapse: The role of pharmacological and behavioral factors'. In O. Pomerleau and C. Pomerleau (eds) *Nicotine Replacement: A Critical Evaluation*. New York: Alan Liss, pp. 163–185.

Stoffregen, T. A. and Riccio, G. E. (1988). 'An ecological theory of orientation and the vestibular system'. *Psychological Review* 95(1), 3–14.

Stopforth, B. (1986). 'Outpatient benzodiazepine withdrawal and the occupational therapist'. *British Journal of Occupational Therapy*, 49(10), 318–322.

Straus, E. (1966). *Phenomenological Psychology*. London: Tavistock Publications.

Stravynski, A. and Greenberg, D. (1987). 'Cognitive therapies with neurotic disorders: clinical utility and related issues'. *Comprehensive Psychiatry* 28(2), 141–150.

Sudnow, D. (1980). *Ways of the Hand*. San Francisco: Jossey Bass.

Summerhoff, G. (1990). 'Life, brain and consciousness'. North Holland: Elsevier. *Consulting and Clinical Psychology* 57(3), 420–424.

Taylor, C. B., Seikh, J., Argas, W. S., Toth, W. T., Margraf, J., Ehlers, A., Maddock, R. J. and Gossard, D. (1986). 'Ambulatory heart rate changes in patients with panic attacks'. *American Journal of Psychiatry* 143, 478–482.

Taylor, C. B., Telch, M. J. and Havvik, D. (1983). 'Ambulatory heart rate changes during panic attacks'. *Journal of Psychiatric Research* 17, 261–266.

Teasdale, J. D. (1983). 'Negative thinking in depression: cause, effect or reciprocal relationship'. *Advances in Behavioural Research and Therapy* 5, 3–25.

Teasdale, J. D. (1993). 'Emotion and two kinds of meaning: cognitive therapy and applied science'. *Behavior Research and Therapy* 31(4), 339–354.

Teasdale, J. D. and Barnard, P. J. (1993). *Affect, Cognition and Change*. Hove: Lawrence Erlbaum.

Tiffany, S. T. (1990). 'A cognitive model of drug urges and drug-use behavior: Role of automatic and nonautomatic processes'. *Psychological Review* 97(2), 147–168.

Tiffany, S. T. and Hakenewerth, D. M. (1991). 'The production of smoking urges through an imagery manipulation: psychophysiological and verbal manifestations'. *Addictive Behaviors* 16, 389–400.

Todd, J. (1957). 'The syndrome of Capgras'. *Psychiatric Quarterly* 31, 250–265.

Trites, R. L. (1969). 'Response sets on the rod and frame test in neurologically impaired subjects'. *Perceptual and Motor Skills* 29, 327–333.

Trueman, D. (1984). 'Depersonalisation in a non-clinical population'. *Journal of Psychology* 116, 107–112.

Turnbull, M. J. and Norris, H. (1982). 'Effects of Transcendental Meditation on self-identity indices and personality'. *British Journal of Psychology* 73, 57–68.

Turner, S. M., Williams, S. L., Beidel, D. C. and Mezzich, J. E. (1986). 'Panic disorder and agoraphobia with panic attacks: covariation along the dimensions of panic and agoraphobic fear'. *Journal of Abnormal Psychology* 95, 384–388.

Tversky, A. and Kahneman, D. (1973). 'Availability: a heuristic for judging frequency and probability'. *Cognitive Psychology* 5, 207–232.

Tyrer, P. (1982). 'Anxiety'. *British Journal of Hospital Medicine* 27, 109–16.

Tyrer, P. and Alexander, J. (1979). 'Classifications of personality disorder'. *British Journal of Psychiatry* 135, 163–167.

Tyrer, P., Owen, R. and Darling, S. (1983). 'Gradual withdrawal of diazepam after long-term therapy'. *Lancet* I, 1402–1406.

Vaillant, G. E. (1983). *The Natural History of Alcoholism: Causes, Patterns and Paths to Recovery*. Cambridge, MA: Harvard University Press.

Van den Hout, M. A. (1988). 'The explanation of experimental panic'. In S. Rachman and J. D. Maser (eds) *Panic: Psychological Perspectives*. London: Erlbaum, pp. 237–253.

Van der Kolk, B. A., Perry, C. and Herman, J. L. (1991). 'Childhood origins of self-destructive behavior'. *American Journal of Psychiatry* 148, 1665–1671.

Velmans, M. (1990). 'Consciousness, brain and the physical world'. *Philosophical Psychology* 3(1), 77–99.

Velten, E. (1968). 'A laboratory task for induction of mood states'. *Behavioural Research and Therapy* 6, 473–482.

Veroff, J., Douvan, E. and Kulka, R. A. (1981). *The Inner American*. New York: Basic Books.

Vojtisek, J. E. (1976). 'Signal detection and size estimation in schizophrenia'. Doctoral dissertation, University of Maine, 1975. *Dissertation Abstracts International* 36, 5290B–5291B (University Microfilms no. 76–7445).

Wachtel, P. L. (1977). *Psychoanalysis and Behaviour Therapy: Towards an Integration*. New York: Basic Books.

Waddel, M. T., Barlow, D. H. and O'Brien, G. T. (1984). 'A preliminary investigation of cognitive and relaxation treatment of panic disorder: effects on intense anxiety versus background anxiety'. *Behaviour Research and Therapy* 22, 393–402.

Walkup, J. (1990). 'On the measurement of delusions'. *British Journal of Medical Psychology* 63, 365–368.

Warr, P. (1982). 'A national study of non-financial employment commitment'. *Journal of Occupational Psychology* 55, 297–312.

Warr, P. (1983). 'Job loss, unemployment and psychological well-being'. In E. van de Vliert and V. Allen (eds) *Role Transitions*. New York: Plenum.

Watts, F. N. (1990). 'New concepts of emotion'. *The Psychologist* 14(2), 75–77.

Watts, F. N. (1992). 'Applications of current cognitive theories of the emotions to the conceptualisation of emotional disorders'. *British Journal of Clinical Psychology* 31, 153–168.

Watts, F. N., Trezise, I. and Sharrock, R. (1986). 'Processing of phobic stimuli'. *British Journal of Clinical Psychology* 25(4), 253–259.

Weaver, C. N. (1980). 'Job satisfaction in the United States in the 1970s'. *Journal of Applied Psychology* 65, 364–367.

Weinberger, D. R. (1984). 'CAT findings in schizophrenia: speculation on the meaning of it all'. *Journal of Psychiatric Research* 18, 477.

Weiner, B. and Graham. S. (1984). 'An attributional approach to emotional development'. In C. E. Izard, J. Kagan and R. B. Zajonc (eds) *Emotions, Cognition and Behaviour*. Cambridge: Cambridge University Press.

Weitzenhoffer, A. M. and Hilgard, E. R. (1962). *Stanford Hypnotic Susceptibility Scale, Form C*. Palo Alto, California: Consulting Psychologists Press.

Werbart, A. (1989). 'Psychotherapy research between process and effect: the need of new methodological approaches'. *Acta Psychiatrica Scandinavica* 79, 511–522.

West, R. and Schneider, N. (1987). 'Craving for cigarettes'. *British Journal of Addiction* 82, 407–415.

West, R. J., Hajek, P. and Belcher, M. (1989). 'Severity of withdrawal symptoms as a predictor of outcome of an attempt to quit smoking'. *Psychological Medicine* 19, 981–985.

White, P. A. (1990). 'Ideas about causation in philosophy and psychology'. *Psychological Bulletin* 108(1), 3–18.

Wiener, M., Budney, S., Wood, L. and Russell, R. L. (1989). 'Nonverbal events in psychotherapy'. *Clinical Psychology Review* 9, 487–504.

Williams, J. M. G., Watts, F. N., MacLeod, C. and Mathews, A. (1988). *Cognitive Psychology and Emotional Disorders*. Chichester: Wiley.

Williams, R. N. (1987). 'Can cognitive psychology offer a meaningful account of meaningful human action?' *The Journal of Mind and Behavior* 8(2), 209–222.

Wilson, T. D. (1990). 'Self-persuasion via self-reflection'. In J. M. Olson and C. L. Hofer (eds) *Self-Inference Processes: Looking Back and Ahead*. London: Methuen.

Witkin, M. A. (1949). 'Perception of body position and of the position of the visual field'. *Psychological Monographs* 6, 7.

Witkin, M. A. (1965). 'Psychological differentiation and forms of pathology'. *Journal of Abnormal Psychology* 70, 317–336.

Witkin, M. A. and Berry, J. W. (1975). 'Psychological differentiation in a cross-cultural perspective'. *Journal of Cross Cultural Psychology* 6, 4–87.

Witkin, M. A. and Goodenough, D. R. (1977). 'Field dependence and interpersonal behavior'. *Psychological Bulletin* 84(4), 661–689.

Wittgenstein, L. (1953). *Philosophische Untersuchungen*. Frankfurt: Suhrkamp Verlag, 1975.

Wittgenstein, L. (1958). *Philosophical Investigations*. Ed. G. E. M. Anscombe. New York: Macmillan.

Woike, B. A. and Aronoff, J. (1992). 'Antecedents of complex social cognitions'. *Journal of Personality and Social Psychology* 63(1), 97–104.

Wolpe, J. (1969). *The Practice of Behavior Therapy*. New York: Pergamon Press.

Woodson, P. P., Buzzi, R. and Battig, K. (1983). 'Effects of smoking on vegetative reactivity to noise'. *Social and Preventative Medicine* 28, 240–241.

Wright, S., Young, A. W, and Hellawell, D. J. (1993). 'Sequential Cotard and Capgras delusions'. *British Journal of Clinical Psychology* 32, 345–349.

Wright, W. F. and Bower, G. H. (1981). 'Mood effects on subjective probability assessment'. Unpublished manuscript, Stanford University.

Yap, P. M. (1965). 'Koro – a culture-bound depersonalization syndrome'. *British Journal of Psychiatry* III, 43–50.

Yardley, L. (1990). 'Motion sickness susceptibility and the utilisation of visual and otolithic information for orientation'. *European Archives of Otorhinolaryngology*.

Young, J. (1990). *Cognitive Therapy for Personality Disorders: a Schema-focused Approach*. Sarasota, FL: Professional Resource Exchange, Inc.

Young, R. Mc. D., Knight, R. G. and Oei, T. P. S. (1990). 'The stability of alcohol-related expectancies in social drinking situations'. *Australian Journal of Psychology* 42(3), 321–330.

Young, R. Mc. D., Oei, T. P. S. and Crook, G. M. (1991). 'Development of a drinking self-efficacy questionnaire'. *Journal of Psychopathology and Behavioral Assessment* 13(1), 1–15.

Zajonc, R. B. (1980). 'Feeling and thinking: preferences need no inferences'. *American Psychologist* 35, 151–175.

Zajonc, R. B. (1984). 'On primacy of affect'. In K. S. Scherer and P. Ekman (eds) *Approaches to Emotion*. Hillsdale, NJ: Lawrence Erlbaum, pp. 247–257.

Zucker, R. A. and Gomberg, E. S. (1986). 'Etiology of alcoholism reconsidered: the case for a biopsychosocial process'. *American Psychologist* 41, 783–805.

Name index

Abed, R.T. 128, 134, 135
Abernathy, E.M. 31
Abernethy, B. 119
Abrams, R. 132, 133
Abse, W. 89
Ackner, B. 92
Afzelius, L. 75
Alexander, J. 111
Alford, B.A. 170–1
Anderson, D.N. 128, 136–7, 139
Anderson, W. 92
Archer, J. 112
Asberg, M. 111
Austin, N. 143
Averill, J.R. 47, 48, 52

Baars, B.J. 20–2, 27
Baddeley, A.D. 31, 174
Baloh, R.W. 78, 81, 82
Bandura, A. 34, 72
Banks, R. 82
Barlow, D.H. 57, 59, 60, 64
Barnard, P.J. 161
Barr, C.C. 82
Beck, A.R. 12, 22, 23, 33–9, *passim*, 43, 44, 48, 58–60 *passim*, 66–72 *passim*, 97, 109, 121, 159, 160, 169–71 *passim*
Bejerot, N. 110
Bellak, I. 80, 97
Bentall, R.P. 28, 139, 169–73 *passim*
Berlyne, N. 132
Berner, P. 55
Berry, J.W. 80
Berson, R.J. 128, 132
Beyts, J. 74, 75, 78, 81
Bidault, E. 132
Binswanger, L. 8–9
Birdwhistell, R.L. 50

Black, F.O. 81
Blackburn, I.M. 37
Bland, K. 70
Bliss, R.E. 111
Bonn, J.A. 62
Borkovec, T.D. 63, 70
Bower, G.H. 29, 30, 32, 36, 51, 160, 161, 169
Bradley, B. 116, 121
Brandt, T. 74, 75, 77, 80
Brentano, F. 4–5
Brett-Jones, J. 167
Brewin, C.R. 165
Brown, R. 113
Brown, S.L. 117
Bullen, J.G. 54
Bullough, E. 152

Callaway, E. 117
Candido, C.L. 54, 169, 170, 172
Capgras, J. 128, 134, 135
Cappon D. 82
Carette, P. 135
Carr, V. 174
Cawthorne, T. 74
Chambless, D.L. 68
Charbonneau, J. 79
Christodoulou, G.N. 127, 130, 132, 136
Churchill, S.C. 178
Clark, D.B. 77
Clark, D.M. 46, 58, 59, 63, 64, 66, 67, 71
Cohen, A.S. 63
Coleman, S.M. 128, 135
Corbit, J.D. 108
Crary, W.G. 76
Craske, M.G. 57, 59, 60, 64
Crichton, P. 127
Csikszentmihalyi, I.S. 147–50 *passim*

Subject index

Milton Keynes UK
Ingram Content Group UK Ltd.
UKHW031148141024
449569UK00024B/962

9 781138 970953